MW01615264

"This is the third bo
"Release Your Obses
share even more pe........ .... from her own
experience and to offer actionable steps for readers.
The Personal Inventory Questions at the end of each
chapter help you reflect on the principles and go
deeper than the usual popular self-help book. If you
are ready to move from being obsessed with your age
– to feeling like you are at your best age ever – then
Dr. Lisa shows you the bridge to heal from the inside
out."
　　　—Mark Stinson, author of A World of Creativity

"In this refreshing new book, Dr.Ortigara Crego
places a positive spin on aging, and reassures the
reader that "age does not define you."

In examples from personal experiences as well as
those from the patients she treats, she shows us how
to approach this last act of our lives. The stark
honesty in admitting her own challenges lends much
credibility to the words she writes. I feel like she's
talking directly to me on these pages, as though we
are having a conversation.

With numerous anecdotes and real current events she
keeps my interest as she proves that age is a mindset.
Like the previous books in this series, she focuses on
a balance of mind, body, and spirit, as she
emphasizes self-care, self-love, and well years rather
than long years.

This book is full of practical advice, and researched up-to-date information, with a touch of humor. I read this book in two days and highly recommend it."

"We're all growing older, and some of us have to face that fact sooner than others. In her latest work of sage, cutting-edge advice, *Release Your Obsession With Aging: Heal from the Inside Out*, Dr. Lisa Ortigara Crego acknowledges it like it is, but also tells readers how much better our stories can be. Taking examples from her decades of therapy practice, she relates individual instances of challenges for older patients and how, together with them, she addressed pressing issues to help them understand and deal with their situations. It's not over until it's over, and we can learn that basic lesson plus lots of not-so-little lessons along the way from Dr. Lisa's latest book. Dr. Lisa is wise and shares her hard-won knowledge to readers' great benefit. This is a lovely book, a helpful book, a valuable book for those of every age, now and in the future."

"Let's face it. The longer we live, the more changes will take place, physically and mentally. This book by Dr. Lisa does not shy away from this fact, and helps us to embrace those changes. The key point she constantly makes is that your mind can either help you or hurt you in the aging process. Again, she uses her own life experiences and those of patients she treated to make her point.

Another well-crafted masterpiece by Dr. Lisa! Not just practical advice for the older generation, but for the younger generation to think ahead about, as they grow older."

— Ed Hendricks, author of Knights of Brave Love

"As am a woman, mom, and psychologist in my mid 40's finding a balance and understanding with the idea of aging gracefully and being able to see the wisdom in my changing body and face Release Your Obsession with Aging: Heal from the Inside Out hits home. Dr. Ortigara Crego offers freedom in her teachings to no longer morph and sculpt ourselves physically. Dr. Ortigara Crego's riveting stories mentally frees us into being our truest selves and live within our most authentic souls."

— Dr. Dara Bushman, psychologist

Release Your Obsession
With Aging

Heal from the Inside Out

Dr. Lisa M. Ortigara Crego

Release Your Obsession with Aging: Heal from the Inside Out
Copyright © 2020 Dr. Lisa Ortigara Crego
EBook ISBN: 978-0-9993025-7-6
Paperback ISBN: 978-0-9993025-6-9
Library of Congress Control Number: 2020947511

The author of this book does not dispense medical advice or prescribe the use of any technique as a form of treatment for physical, emotional, or medical problems without the advice of a physician, either directly or indirectly. The intent of the author is only to offer information of a general nature to help you in your quest for emotional, spiritual, and physical well-being. In the event you use any of the information in this book for yourself, which is your constitutional right, the author and the publisher assume no responsibility for your actions.

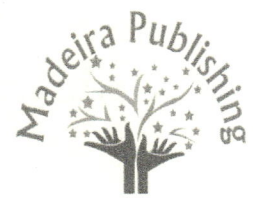

Madeira Publishing
Hollywood, Florida
Madeirapublising.com

MEDICAL DISCLAIMER

DEDICATION

*Dedicated to all those chasing youth,
that you may find your inward beauty,
in order to beam your exterior beauty.*

FOREWORD

Imagine if you will, receiving guidance and answers to resolve difficulties you may be having in body, mind, or spirit…all in one place.

Well here it is: how to replace many faulty beliefs about aging being a time of decline. When you know what to do, you will find that aging can be a period of growth and purpose.

I had the exquisite pleasure of being able to take a peek at this timely and powerful book: *Release Your Obsession With Aging*: *Heal from the Inside out,* right before its publication.

What I found is that the author, **Dr. Lisa Ortigara Crego,** is turning entrenched "human race-consciousness beliefs" about aging upside down. It is Dr. Lisa and people like her who are breaking up the calcified opinions that have been passed down to us for generations about aging. She stands her ground while she encourages us to not go back to sleep. She implores us to step out of our conditioning and faulty ideas about the aging process. You know, the kind of persuasive, erroneous beliefs, which circulate that after 40 it's all downhill from there. Convictions that allocate the boxes we should be checking as each decade passes—such as becoming invisible as we grow older, and the feeling that if we are seen, at least keep quiet.

Dr. Lisa makes clear, based on her personal experience of healing her own earlier obsessions, professionally helping clients for many years, and well-backed research that if we don't change stereotypical thinking, we will view the aging process negatively. We won't be able to see aging as a time of boundless mysteries and wisdom but more or less an enemy that we have to fight.

We are as delusional as Don Quixote flaying at windmills when we distract ourselves, believing that we can fight the inevitable. Acceptance is the beginning of our process, and the author gives us many permissions or starting points encouraging us to begin where we are, not where we think we should be. For instance, when I look in the mirror, I may not like my aging body, but I am grateful for it and all that it does for me. Note the small shift in energy toward myself that starts the day on a better note.

Dr. Lisa Ortigara Crego also acknowledges that acceptance does not mean we like the idea of aging, but we have to create a new foundation in which to hold our changes.

The crossing of the threshold into later years is a time when one can be very happy. I personally attest to all Dr. Lisa says. I am a happy older person, much happier now than during the first 50 years of my life. People like me who enjoy their later years generally have in common a deep love, passion, or commitment to a cause that is bigger than our little personal selves. This is the Spiritual Depth that the author emphasizes. I do my little bit to alter, where I can, the world's inequality through helping Womankind... I passionately encourage women to stand up and be counted and claim their rightful place in the world.

No black balloons here

Dr. Lisa clarifies, identifies, and encourages us to ask the right questions, to accept the tools and guidance she offers so we can break out of the boxes allocated for older people. We can actually be joyful in our later years when we release limiting beliefs.

Dr. Lisa offers a lot of understanding and compassion for our "stuckness," which calls for deep "vertical" healing. This is not your usual horizontal type change. You know, when we become frenetically busy; buy new makeup; shop for new clothes; maybe even change jobs or houses—just surface modifications. Not here. This work about aging and the difficulties we have with it in our culture addresses the necessity of a seismic amendment.

This excellent work can only come from the heart and pen of one who has overcome relentless obstacles that others might consider impossible to breach. No matter what has us by the scruff of the neck about aging, she gives us hope and permission, inner and outer, to activate more of our hidden courage, determination, and resilience

Dr. Lisa Ortigara Crego shows us a range of ways to let go of discouragement, anxiety, depression, and self-deprecation. She shares her personal journey and gives us many case studies that illuminate the difficulties of exposing hidden root causes. She explains the importance of reflection and a thorough inventory, a decision to come out of denial and no longer wait. Our time to change beliefs that keep us unhappy is now.

I am particularly excited about Dr. Lisa's new book as a wonderful resource to recommend to my clients, both men and women. As one who has practiced psychotherapy for over 30 years, specializing in issues that touch women of all ages, I know how difficult the aging process can be. I also know that we make it more difficult if we accept the usual beliefs and myths

If you dare read this book and practice the powerful ways of uncovering and healing hidden and faulty beliefs, you will never be able to return to what you thought you knew about aging. As all good books have the power to do, this one will turn everything you thought you knew around, making space for new beginnings and happiness that you never expected. And so it is!

Laura B. Young MS. LMFT. CCH.

Author of…

Remove Obstacles to Experience Unstoppable Feminine Power: How to Stop Betraying Yourself and Life a Life of Grace and Passion

http://FemininePowerBooks.com

https://www.laurabyoung.com

Introduction

Stir Up The Gift Of God Which Is In You.
~2 Timothy 1:6

Life would be much simpler if we were all born with a book that told us how to age gracefully, a book that answered our deepest internal fears and gave us the go-ahead that it's okay to age, a book that delivered support when we needed it. But in the end, we must all write this book for ourselves and find our true path in life, as it unfolds.

That we will age is inevitable, and we will all die, but we can embrace the journey—or not. *Stir up the gift of God, which is in you.* This gift is in each of us—it is not the outside that speaks to our soul—our inner being—but rather what is within.

One day, in the spring of 1998 I attended a workshop at the Diplomat hotel near Miami, Florida with many influential speakers such as Brian Weiss and James Van Praagh, and a host of others I don't recall.

This came but a few months after my best friend, Yvonne, unexpectedly passed away in her sleep. My mom had a massive stroke on the eve of the eve before Easter; my son's grandpa died from cancer; my husband's father's car crashed, cascading over the side of a mountain in Puerto Rico, plunging my father-in-law to his death.

What prompted me to go to this particular workshop was just the nudge I needed. On a brisk winter day for South Florida, I trudged into one of the Weight Watchers centers where I was to give a lecture on food and inner strength, though I surely wasn't feeling it.

My head hung low, I barely made eye contact with members — or staff for that matter. I hurt. I was questioning life, yet pushing through to help others. But why bother with such a positive outlook? So we can age and then die?

No, I wasn't feelin' it that day. I felt sad, alone, engulfed in grief over the recent losses. Each one was an untimely shocker, and all those around me were losing loved ones too.

Mandy, one of the greeters at the front, welcomed me with her warm smile, noting I wasn't my usual upbeat self. After prodding, I shared my sorrows. She stopped me midstream, marched out of the lobby area, out of the center itself, and briskly made her way to her car trunk.

Watching Mandy's head buried deep in the belly of the large trunk from the picture window, I saw that she was franticly pulling out this and that — quite a stash, in fact, until she retrieved a perfectly crisp newspaper, which upon her return she thrust into my hands, saying, "Read this — you'll feel better."

I nonchalantly crammed it into my briefcase, barely giving it a glance, mumbling my thanks and then pressed on with my lecture. I forgot the newspaper until a few days later when I stumbled over it lying on the floor of my car.

I hadn't even looked at it.

I flipped through the pages to find an article about this man, Brian L. Weiss, who at the time was chief of psychiatry at Mount Sinai Medical Center in Miami Beach, Florida.

Apparently while practicing psychotherapy/hypnotherapy, Dr. Weiss had encountered Catherine, a twenty-seven-year-old woman with major anxiety issues, depression, and a wide array of phobias. She worked as a lab tech at the same hospital.

The experience with Catherine led him to write, *Many Lives Many Masters: The True Story of a Prominent Psychiatrist, His Young Patient, and the Past-Life Therapy That Changed Both Their Lives* in 1988. I was intrigued, especially because I too was conducting hypnosis, though not Weiss's type of regression therapy but rather the here-and-now sort, removing fears, anxiety, and habits.

I pored over the article, not once, but several times. I was amazed. The piece discussed Dr. Weiss's journey from disbelief to belief in regard to both messages from the supernatural world and reincarnation.

As a practicing Catholic, I wasn't convinced of past life claims, since that seemed a bit farfetched — and the psychiatrist, too, had his doubts, until he regressed Catherine to discuss experiences she couldn't possibly have known in *this* life. She also went on talking about the doctor's loss of his firstborn baby, along with other personal information, *that he'd not told anyone.*

I felt some sense of hope for Yvonne and all my loved ones, that perhaps they weren't so far away — that perhaps death wasn't the end. So I ventured off to the newspaper office to ask the attendant for several copies, as I thought to share them with others hurting from their loss.

After scanning the front of the article, the handsome young man from India said, "Ma'am, this article is very old...ten years old to be exact." And it surely was. I was shocked. It was crisp and clean — and yet it had been in Mandy's disarrayed, overstuffed, trunk for ten years. *Ten years.* Oh my, and here when I needed to read such a piece she'd pulled it out — in 1998 — after all my tragic losses.

I had never read anything like this before — nor had I personally experienced so many lives lost at the same time.

It Was Meant To Be

So when I learned a few weeks later that the very author, Dr. Brian Weiss, was presenting at the Diplomat in Miami, I *had* to go. I yearned to hear his story. I purposely went alone to soak it in. After his riveting two-hour talk — partly with James Van Praagh, an American psychic — I met with Dr. Weis alone for a few minutes.

Dr. Weiss was true to his themes, which included: spiritual conversion; connection with the dead; and the importance of universal religious teachings such as concerning charity, faith, and love. He was warm and welcoming of my questions, and humble in the face of my awe.

Dr. Weiss was no slump. He had been classically trained at Columbia University and Yale Medial School, graduating with many honors. The psychiatrist himself admitted to being the last person in the world open to channeling, reincarnation, and parapsychology.

Now please know this is *not* a book about psychics and spiritual phenomena, but more about life's challenges and unexpected experiences as you power through the aging process.

Life unveils many hidden treasures when we least expect them—*when we need them*. I was searching for signs that more than the here and now existed—that we had connections to the beyond—that life had so many miracles yet waiting for me in spite of these tragic events.

And—so it was true—more awaits us.

I had come to the workshop because of the difficulties I was having as a clinician—not knowing anything in this arena because of my inadequate training in life's tragedies and losses. At that point in my career, I was involved in extensive training covering dealing with patients' eating disorders, addictions, and losses. I was just scratching the surface of psychotherapy, all while working on my own issues of binge eating disorder, food addiction, bulimia through over-exercising, and *very* low self-esteem. This was, in fact, during my own early but shaky weight loss of one hundred pounds, which I'd lost and gained back several times before.

At that time, I was interning at Sylvester Cancer Center, working with people who were at the end-stage of their cancers. Aging and dying were around me at every turn, and I was searching for answers as to how to beat this weight issue once and for all...and to show others the way.

I also had worked for Weight Watchers of Greater Miami for nearly ten years as a lecturer, where I remained another three years after I was freshly graduated in 1996. So I was a babe in the woods, with much to learn.

Body, Mind, and Spirit

Like many psychotherapists, I had built walls around myself as protection from the emotional pain I was personally feeling and seeing in patients as well. My training was in how to treat mental illness as it related to many psychological issues, particularly eating disorders, mood disorders, and addictions. I wanted to take this work a step further and treat the whole self: body, mind, and spirit.

I wanted to treat the *whole* person—and myself, additionally. I thought I was supposed to have all the answers—and when I didn't, I began to feel like a failure.

Around the same time, I began to read Bernie Siegel, M.D.'s book, *How to Live Between Office Visits*, at which exposure, I began to understand that I wasn't alone in feeling this inadequacy, and that as we practice we gain insights.

"I know now that we teach what we need to learn," wrote Dr. Siegel. I heard this message over and over from others who had walked before me in the helping industry. And so, now I'm teaching about aging as I'm powering my way through that process, as well.

Dr. Siegel went on to say, "I'm sure I was sensing a need in myself to learn how to live too." His words sparked an awakening within me, with the same need.

More than twenty-two years after that eye-opening workshop, I'm privileged to make my living teaching thousands of people—men and women, young and old—how to live their best lives through self-love, self-care, and spiritual awareness so they can heal from the inside out.

In addition, when you strip away the processed foods; learn how to eat whole, rich foods with nutrients; and spend on quality foods rather than fast foods, you'll have an abundance of health bonuses, one being slowing down the aging process and maybe even beating some of the standard diseases out there such as diabetes, heart disease, anxiety, etc.

I wrote my first three books on obsession with food, mind chatter, and cheat days respectively. I thought I'd covered what I needed to say, but, once again, my work was not done. Day in and day out, I watched patients chasing youth—*and it starts early.* Some are only in their thirties and they're shooting up

Botox as if it's heroin. Or they're going for rhinoplasty, butt lifts, breast and lip augmentation — and the list goes on.

I'm not saying plastic surgery is a bad thing, because surely it's not. But what I am saying is such procedures can become an obsession and out of control — as you'll see in the pages ahead. But you'll also note how many find *their happy place* exactly where they are as they reach toward self-actualization.

I discovered that a vast number of patients with eating disorders, if not all, had body image challenges lurking in the background. And with body image often come weight obsessions and body part obsessions — and eventually age obsession, trailing close behind.

My goal here is to lead you to a healthy relationship with your body, touching on weight and eating disorders as I thread through the issue of fear of aging. By the time you finish this book, you'll feel confident regarding what is right and what is not right for you. I promise.

I've helped patients and readers alike with weight issues, body image, diet obsessions, and food addiction, and now I'd like to help you live free from the obsession with aging.

Feel the Fear — And Do It Anyway

Aging gracefully. Stop and envision what you would feel like being at peace and not plagued by the obsession with aging — knowing that for once you have no urge to lean into the mirror and count every new line—every new sag, wrinkle, bump, vein, or newly popped-up something. I promise if you look close enough you *will* find something, I know I do.

What would you feel like to master and work through what you're afraid of as you allow yourself to age with dignity and honor? Perhaps you have fears over pending illnesses or seeing others you love aging and becoming frail, or worse, approaching death, and you fear this will happen to you, too. And it might—but chances are it won't and certainly not in the same way or at the same time as you imagine. So, spending precious moments focusing on the might ofs and should ofs and could ofs is squandering unrecoverable time.

As we age, we're entering the unknown—all of us. We don't know what to expect on any given day, and perhaps others' misfortunes create obsessions and fears concerning our own forecasts.

When we embed another's misfortunes as a possibility that they could be ours, we begin to fester with the worry—the obsession. If we stay in the now and embrace our good fortune, take care of ourselves with healthful nutrition, moderate exercise, and daily grooming and hygiene—particularly in relation to our teeth—we are on our way to aging gracefully.

Perhaps you're chasing diets and wanting to become thin, believing that would bring back youth and postpone aging. And maybe it will. I'm not saying don't look your best and be your fittest. But what I am saying is stop the insane nonsense in your head pushing you to look 20 when you're 50.

One woman I saw years back, Jana, was 80-something, engaged in enough plastic surgery to create a thirty-year-old face. She had surgery upon surgery to sculpt the most gorgeous young face possible.

Now you might think, *What's wrong with that?* Well, our hands, gait, voice, and necks can't be 30. Seeing the mismatch might seem creepy. Nothing is wrong with bettering the self, even if that means working in a cosmetic surgery or two, or even three. That's up to you — a personal decision. It's okay. What's not okay is when the surgery becomes obsessive (does Michael Jackson come to mind?) or when in the aging process you become gripped with terror of the next line, sag, or aging something.

Signs of aging are going to happen — *to all of us*, in time, if we live long enough. But we can go through the changes with open arms, while taking care along the way to preserve and promote good health from the inside out — and the goal of this book is to encourage that.

A Nip, Tuck, and Cream?

What would you feel like going anywhere at any time with anyone, harboring no worries about how to present yourself as youthful — or better yet, being satisfied with exactly who you are, as you are, *as you look now*. To no longer use plastic surgeries, Botox, or even expensive creams as your fast track (back) to youth or as an indulgence in achieving whatever you want—or whatever deals you've made with yourself.

Again, you will find phenomenal products out there and surgeries that can make a difference in a positive way, but you may also trip across marketing geniuses who want you as a customer, client, or patient—and who suck you in with promises. To that point, I opened an email recently entitled, "Crepe Erase." The wording went on to say: *"Finally! Treat Your Age-Giveaway Zones* with an amazing product from this Hollywood actress—the astonishing SECRET to younger-looking skin. Order now."

Hmm, I thought. I don't know for a fact, but I'd guess the actress shown eats healthfully, exercises, takes impeccable care of her teeth, doesn't drug or drink, and lives her full best life. Sure, *Crepe Erase* may help but this nearly 70-year-old most likely was lovely from the start. The ad is pulling people like you, and me, in—making a promise—perhaps that we can look like the lovely woman we've seen on TV.

Yes, you—the obsessed with aging you (myself included) are who the marketers target. Promises are made that sound *so* good. These experts, a team of psychologists, doctors, marketers, scientists, and others work on our emotions in a thirty-second email or commercial clip. They've gotta reel you in, *fast*. They'll sell you a burnt-out light bulb, convincing you if you rub it on your skin you'll radiate. Okay, don't try that…

No doubt death and aging are looming for all of us. As some say, "We're not going to get out of this alive." Sure, that's a bit daunting, and maybe even scary, but it's true. So use your time here on planet earth wisely. You don't have to look haggard and old, but you also don't have to obsess over every product promise that pops up. Start with the basics and let that lead you...

Maybe you fear your own transition from this life, or how it will pan out. But what if you filled your time with productive, on-purpose, and on-point experiences, and lived to the very best of your ability? Perhaps then, when you take that last breath, you can smile and say, "It was good." Often the fear that is prompting the obsession is far worse than the reality.

Maybe you're trying to slow the ticking clock. I recall when I was twenty-nine and staring down the clock as it was about to strike midnight, and I no longer would be in my twenties. I was terrified. My heart was pounding as it clicked to each succeeding second, watching the small hand make its way around the clock. Try as I might, I couldn't will that clock to stop ticking. I turned thirty.

That night, more than half my life ago, was the only time I ever recall fearing the numbers turning. When I was twelve years old, I rushed the time to become a teenager. With my heart beating fast at the exhilaration of turning a number older, I could barely stand to wait. The small hand couldn't move fast enough. Ahh, the sound of thirteen was super cool to me. Perhaps that's the attitude we need now...no more fearing the turning of the dial, instead embrace it *and you will find youth.*

You Are Not Your Age

Laura B. Young, author of *Remove Obstacles to Experience Unstoppable Feminine Power: How to Stop Betraying Yourself and Live a Life of Grace and Passion*, writes, "Remember none of us are the age we look." I love that line. Think about it, none of us are the age we look.

I recall years back a close friend, Susan, nearing sixty, told me just that, but in different words. "I know I'm getting older, but inside I feel exactly the same as always in my thoughts and in my inner world." I thought, *How interesting to still be the same you inside but look older on the outside.*

Today, I'm the age she was all those years ago, and she was right, totally right. I don't feel my age inside. I still think the same in the inner world of my mind — just as I did in my youth. *We are not our age.*

Your social status does not define you, either. Nor does your body define you. Your money doesn't define you. Your business doesn't define you. No — only your authentic you defines you.

The Promise

No book, psychologist, psychotherapist, spiritualist, or life coach can guarantee that your out-of-control obsession with aging will cease for the rest of your life, or that you will always feel fantastic without aches and pains, just as no one can guarantee you will live to one hundred without a taint of issues — or that you will live life in perfect harmony every single minute of the coming time without a hiccup — even if you live in the best of situations.

But I can promise to show you ways to maneuver through life's ups and downs no matter the transition through stages we all will greet as we move on through our years, if you practice the suggestions laid out in this book. As you power through these pages, you will master your changes without fear or obsession. You will live your best life from the inside out.

By the time you finish reading *Release Your Obsession With Aging: Heal from the Inside Out*, you will be able to skillfully arrest any inner or outer turmoil focused on the one wrinkle or sag or bump — which can morph into terrific anxiety as you try to stop the clock. But instead, for once, you will live free from the burdens and fears of what ifs, no longer white knuckling and forcing change in an unnatural way.

You will no longer live for your younger days but rather embrace the maturity at each level as it unveils. You will have collected an arsenal of strategies to silence the fear of the unknown, and once and for all free yourself from the burdens you have entrapped in your unreasonable *must-be-young* mentality.

Explorations

I have set up this book, as I do all of my books, to take you through a series of explorations, just the way I would if you came to me weekly as a private patient for psychotherapy, sharing positive and negative experiences from my own life and the lives of others who walked this path prior to, during, and after recovery. The book opens with my story followed by a discussion and understanding of *Aging — The Obsession*, unpacking the *what* and *why* as they're wrapped around a *young-is-in and old-is-out* mentality.

My goal is to show you how to release obsessive, negative, self-destructive self-and body-image connections and build a confident you on all occasions, whether age and weight is involved or not. My goal is to remove the youth-as-the-center-of-your-universe attitude and replace it with positive self-reflection as your lifeline, no matter your current age placement, whether twenty or ninety and everything in between.

Along with an attempt to reveal how I have come to grips with the incessant *gotta-stay-young* mentality, I also endeavor to help readers meet this difficult challenge through practical, structured, step-by-step, synthesized information and advice, including anecdotes to demonstrate how individuals may obtain relief and resolution of never-ending issues arising from destructive thinking and behavior as it relates to the process of winding down or winding up in life.

As you weave through the chapters, you will encounter discussions as to why the fear of getting old, with the intention of fighting it tooth and nail, become your primary focus rather than the journey itself. I'll discuss how obsessive thinking leads to a frantic goal of fighting the aging process—unnaturally. And you'll be led to examine how questions of food, drink, and body size take up residence in your activities, as you grow older.

Because the pandemic of COVID-19 sprouted in the middle of my writing this book, that topic intrudes and weaves throughout the pages as it relates to aging, and all that comes with it.

Moreover, a book on *aging* that shows up as an obsession would be missing the mark if the topics of certain deteriorations were ignored, such as: worries over illness, fear of death, or the onslaught of new wrinkles, or the unexpected drop of this or that caused by gravity, and not to mention surgeries. Further, then we have to consider food and diets, with the expectation of many that thin means young. But does it?

Maybe you wonder what body weight has to do with the process of aging or genetics versus your lifestyle, or maybe how human growth hormone fits into the mix—all of these areas seem to contribute to the march toward young, while age continues to add up.

But not to worry, realignment sorts through the process making sense of it all as you move through and away from the obsession—to start healing from the inside out.

From *Aging—The Obsession* we continue into *Realignment,* which is the positive development of self, the advancement through the upheaval—the shift and renewal of your best you as you transition away from the obsession to a productive, happy, free-spirited self.

What can you do to alter the aging process? Should you sit idle and let time pass without any contribution toward an optimal life no matter the age? NO, absolutely not. This is about realigning your thinking and behavior, to move away from the fear-grip of aging to the grace-grip, so you can embrace life, whether your introvert or extrovert life calls. And yes, you want to live exactly where you are within yourself but as your *best self* because age does not define you. The goal is to reach your pinnacle of self-actualization.

Working through and realigning using a bag of tools such as authenticity is an excellent starting place. Mixed in with the realigning phase, a major imperative is to have a new relationship with foods, understanding how to put together a healthy meal — which foods are good for you, and which are age sapping. I encourage readers toward a whole-body approach: body, mind, and spirit

How, you ask? First you must start from where you are and love you with the beautiful blessing bestowed on you. Give thanks for your eyes to see, ears to hear, arms to hug, and legs to stand strong on, and then, as you venture out, you will embrace all situations age related. This is an opportunity for you to reset, but with more vigor; you are decked with wisdom beyond that possessed by youth.

As you become more at ease, you'll handle twists and turns during scary times such as surgery, disease, or skin cancer. You'll be armed and ready to embrace life as it unfolds.

The chapters also unpack the importance of understanding and employing each tool on the journey of recovery from obsessive, inner, negative conversations such as, "but my face is changing," or an "I will miss out if I don't join the needle Botox gang or have surgeries" kind of thought (and action) process.

As the realignment unfolds, the chapters explore food addiction and aging along with nutrition, mood, energy, and wrinkles. Eating quality, non-processed foods is the perfect start to healing the body—*inside and out*. Real food is the key to ignite optimism and lessen anxiety, enhance energy, clear the skin, and provide an overall sense of wellbeing, not to mention slow the aging process. All of these are tied together—*you'll see*. But we can discover a way out. I promise.

From **Realignment** you'll **Turn The Corner** where change takes hold, the kind of change that you embrace with pride wherever you are in your life's journey. In this phase, you'll recognize that little efforts go a long way. As you turn the corner with movement, not just exercise but movement, you will *feel* something happening.

The age-old saying, "The more you do, the more you can do" is true. Our bodies become crusty, stiff, rigid, and unbending, when we sit without doing. This process is about moving, walking with nature, opening up your "God" connection, and becoming reacquainted with your spiritual self.

Turning the corner is about looking at retirement—or not—through a new lens. It's about *imagining* your later years into reality. Let's face it; we all need something to look forward to, no matter the age or chapter in our lives. The advice is not to give up, not now, not ever—but to take that last breath with a smile on your lips, knowing your trip through life was good—you did good.

The most important message as you turn the corner is to recognize and rehearse one reality in your thoughts over and over: Age does not define you.

At this juncture, you move into areas that bring you great joy—like the relationship with others. People need others, whether friends, lovers, children, babies, or puppies, along with any further stripe of fur and feather buddies you prefer.

In addition, you'll find the chapters here speckled with words of self-care, self-love, and spiritual fueling, as these are the foundation of your wellbeing and the gateway to your highest hierarchy of need.

And it goes without saying that throughout the chapters you'll be coached to move away from a standard American diet (SAD)—which is both sad (for your body) and costly—and encouraged to move toward a healthful American diet wherein you spend less money while eating better-quality foods.

And of course, we will examine working through the emotional component that comes with the promise of *releasing your obsession with aging* as we turn another year older, and how the fretting can be rerouted to gratitude for breath and appreciation for our lives. We will look at how every day can be a good day, from start to finish. All pathways to releasing your obsessions with aging are incorporated into this book.

If you will examine your personal inventory as questions appear following each chapter and practice the golden nuggets scattered throughout the pages, by the time you reach the end of this material, you will have begun to change your life.

My immediate goal is to help you release your obsession with negative aging ideation and connect to a better you in twenty-one days or less, thanks to:

✓ The book's groundbreaking identification of the *what* and the *why* of believing *aging* is the culprit — that youth will *complete* you.
✓ The incorporation of easy, step-by-step customizable day-to-day "outpatient" actions to help you navigate through the jungle of treatments, serums, surgeries, and old belief systems from childhood or cultural connections that advancing age is NOT a good thing.
✓ Personal Inventory Questions throughout, designed to identify and reprogram your aging mentality and open your unique natural/spiritual path to recovery.

My suggestion is that you first read through the book once to orient yourself to this approach. Then you can slowly read the book again—only this time working through the questions following the end of each chapter.

As you read, you'll also note that every chapter opens with an inspirational quote from a spiritual leader, author, or the Bible. Don't skip these valuable morsels of wisdom, as they're real treasures, designed to start you thinking at a deeper level.

Why Another Book On Obsession

Often, while writing this, I have been asked how this book ever came into being. I think the best answer is that after I wrote my first book, *Release Your Obsession with Food: Heal from the Inside Out*, I realized my work wasn't done but rather only beginning. To unravel and correct eating disorders takes tapping into the many realms of releasing your obsession with food, leading to my second book, *Release Your Obsession with Diet Chatter*, drilling into the topic of obsessive thoughts about food and diets—which led to the third book, *Release Your Obsession with Cheat DAZE*, looking into the lies we tell ourselves in adopting a cheat day mentality.

I needed to lead those in trouble with food addiction away from the grip of their compulsion to the refuge of eating recovery, from negative inner chatter to positive inner considerations, to disbanding the *cheat day* mentality by eating healthful foods no matter *where you are* or *who you are with*, no matter the occasion.

The latter, of course, is what blossomed into this fourth book—how to **Release Your Obsession With Aging** so that you can continue to heal from the inside out—because the obsessions don't end with food, relentless thoughts, and cheat days; often they move on to an attempt to defy aging by what can be extreme and expensive measures. My goal here then is to help you move away from any makeshift elaboration you have conjured up in your belief system that hooks into a negative would-be age-defying mentality.

I have no doubt that being young provides a fun and exciting whirl of emotions and activities—but all phases of our lives have their time and season. This is not to say we shouldn't stay youthful, because we should, but not to the point of indulging a gripping obsession.

You see, we become attached to ideas and never let them go, creating a reference system that turns into our way of thinking, behaving, and acting out. Just like Jana, mentioned earlier, who wanted to be young to such an extent that she took every opportunity to create a young face on her very aged body. She struggled with aging gracefully, as she believed she couldn't be her authentic self if she didn't have the look of youth.

Jana searched high and low in every magazine and Internet advertisement and on billboard images in an obsessed quest to regain her youth. All the doctors knew of Jana, and sadly they welcomed her time and time again, joining her journey of defying age, and knowing she was suffering psychologically and that each procedure was hurting her more emotionally, physically, and financially.

Jana believed she wouldn't have the *right look* if she didn't dive into the next best procedure — making *looking* young the center of her being rather than *feeling* young. She missed the here and now as she was in her head obsessing over whether she looked young enough.

Jana hunted down wrinkles or growths, studying her face in a well-lit magnified mirror rather than smiling back at the natural twinkle in her crisp blue eyes. Such a pattern could only cloud any opportunity to bathe in the love of self and connections with others.

That said, Jana also suffered from binge-eating disorder with a long, long history of dieting and bingeing, followed by more dieting and more bingeing. On any given day, she might carry an additional forty pounds, which was her "set-point," the weight her body tended to align to.

In time, Jana learned to break the negative pattern, and she was able to move in a positive direction. She began to experience her aging with love and openness, while eating the healthy versions of food, losing any and all self-degradation, replacing that with self-acceptance.

Please note that eating disorders, mental illnesses, mood disorders, and addictions are serious and often require a village to conquer. You owe it to yourself to tap into a pool of help, such as through psychotherapy, group therapy, sessions with a psychiatrist, and/or time spent in places of worship with reference to your spiritual connection. Twelve-step meetings, books on these topics, and any other mode of help that fits your needs and preferences are definitely recommended.

Jana chose psychotherapy, hypnotherapy, and meditation, along with any and all spiritual practices to work on her addiction to cosmetic surgeries, binge eating, and addictive obsessions with sugar, flour, and wheat. She now continues to reach for self-actualization — the fulfillment and recognition of her talents and potentialities.

Where to Begin...

To start the process of healing your thoughts and behaviors, begin with self-love and self-care. The essence of what frees us away from the obsessive self-scrutiny is love. You can learn to love your face and body as it is now and move away from fad surgery promises of youth into a natural life journey — to heal your body and heal your mind — *from the inside out*.

Americans are caught up in defying aging, death denial, dieting to look young, accessing products that make false promises. We can't stop chasing the fads, the get-young-quick-schemes, hoping that THIS TIME we'll break free from out-of-control thinking while body obsessing and longing for a youthful fix.

And yet, at the same time, the age-defying quest is consuming our thoughts: when to Botox or nip and tuck, and what creams will *youthenize* — with promises that we hope will fill our sadness, lift our spirits, and bring unrealistic assurances to fruition.

A conditioning from the past says that youth is in, old is out. I learned this as a small child hearing my father lament about turning mid-thirties, or while watching television and hearing my dad say, "Oh, Joan, look how old so and so looks" as if we're not supposed to age. I felt his words as saying aging is disgusting. Or I'd hear about this one or that one dying or getting old or sick or anything that showed abhorrence of the very idea of aging — a perfectly normal process.

The patients and people discussed in *Release Your Obsession With Aging* range from individuals in their later teens and mid-twenties into adulthood, all the way to nineties and above — transitioning to the end of life. All those mentioned in the book were acquaintances, people associated with twelve-step groups, and/or those in psychotherapy. Many passed away years back.

In accordance with twelve-step protocol and patient confidentiality, names have been changed and at times genders, nationalities, hair, and looks in general were switched to keep each person, including acquaintances, anonymous. Often a person mentioned is a combination of several persons, all harboring similar issues and backgrounds.

This is a book about getting out of your own way with aging in order to become your true, authentic spiritual self without going into a swirl of obsessions over the natural process of getting older.

If you're looking for something easy or fast, though, you have the wrong book. If you're looking for a book to help you become young in a nanosecond without effort, you have the wrong book. If you're looking for a medical guru to explain in depth the ins and outs of nutrition and cosmetic surgeries, you have the wrong book.

But if you're looking for a book to lead you out of the self-degrading hunt for youth, no matter your age—a freedom beyond your wildest expectations, *long term*—this is the book for you. If you're looking to reach self-actualization—your highest spiritual self, you've found it.

Dave Ramsey in his *The Total Money Makeover* says, "IF YOU LIVE LIKE NO ONE ELSE, LATER YOU CAN LIVE LIKE NO ONE ELSE." I love this quote because it applies to so many areas in addition to your becoming debt free. Though this book is not a total money makeover, it is a total "youth makeover," *in the natural way,* of course.

No gimmicks, bells or whistles here. I say, "If you youth like no one else, later you can youth like no one else," meaning you will learn *your* personal plan that works for you with living your authentic life and not letting age define you. You will learn to reset food, mood, and wrinkles without pressing "gotta get young, can't age" buttons. .

This book is written to suggest techniques and to give examples demonstrating YOU don't need to be defeated by anything, that you can have peace of mind, improved health, and a never-ceasing flow of energy—at any age. This book is to steer you from chasing youth to chasing your best life in the here and now.

Release Your Obsession with Aging: Heal from the Inside Out is for anyone trying to end the obsession with aging. The goal is to end the pursuit after every age-defying product out there and lead you to heal from the inside out as I practice with the first three books.

I learned firsthand and now I'm passing it along to you…

Table of Contents

Part I

Aging - The Obsession

Chapter 1

My Story

*Taking care is the one way
to show your love.
~Fred Rogers*

Though Fred Rogers was a master at *feeling* children's feelings, which was how he was able to reach them, he also crafted many wise words we adults could learn a thing or two from as well. Self-care and self-love are paramount to aging gracefully, so that we can live full, healthy lives. I didn't get that until my mid-adult life, but get it I did—and so will you.

Maybe you were taught at a young age that if you cared for yourself you were being selfish—a message that can be confusing, often creating guilt within. Living a full and healthy life requires attention to your self-needs, by you or someone who loves you, if you can't care for yourself. Living a full and healthy life doesn't mean you'll live a long life, but it does mean you'll up your chances significantly of living your best life while here.

Living a long life is often the goal, but think about increasing the span of healthy life as your more important goal. Rather than striving for a longer life, how about trying to increase your number of well years. What is a well year? It's a year of complete wellness, or a year of life free of dysfunction, symptoms, and health-related problems. It's living as a whole you, body, mind, and spirit.

And self-actualization is what we strive for to become our authentic selves. As a college professor, I taught the concept of psychologist Abraham Maslow's hierarchy of needs, which points to individuals reaching their full potential. Students always thought that meant having enough money...but actually it means reaching your authentic self at a spiritual level—a want-for-nothing stage. It means reaching one's potential and one's self-fulfillment.

Maslow's pyramid starts with basic physiological needs such as food, water, warmth, and rest. Moving up a rung of the ladder, we come to safety and security, then followed by love and belonging, where intimate relationships and friendships are developed. The next rung finds us at esteem needs such as prestige and feelings of accomplishment. Last comes self-actualization, which means achieving one's full potential, including in creative activities. This last self-fulfillment is the place you want to reach, as it's the pinnacle of life, the situation where you can exhale and say, "It was good."

My Life

My own independent life began very early. By twelve, I was fending for myself for most of my needs. I barely had the food, water, warmth, and rest marking the early rungs of the ladder because I found myself reaching to fulfill my needs so early on. Mom was showing German shepherds all around the country while Dad traveled between houses, and all my siblings left home young, leaving me to care for myself. Most times, I didn't feel secure, and I didn't feel safe. I was alone; hence, my eating disorders began.

I'm not saying I was abused or that I had this horrible childhood, for I did not. Rather, I had a permissive, negligent mom and an absent father, which meant I had to figure out how to handle the basics early in life. I know Mom and Dad did the best they could from where they were at that time. I love them both with my heart and soul—may they rest in peace.

A Beautiful Day in the Neighborhood

I was gifted *A Beautiful Day in the Neighborhood: Neighborly Words of Wisdom from Mister Rogers* this past holiday season and recently began reading. In the opening, "Can You Say...Hero?" by Tom Junod, he eloquently notes Mr. Rogers weighed 143 pounds. He always weighed 143 pounds. And Junod goes on to say that Mr. Rogers refused to do anything to rattle that weight.

Mr. Rogers neither drank, smoked, nor ate flesh of any kind, nor went to bed late, nor slept in, nor watched television—but he did swim every morning. Mr. Rogers came to see the number 143 as a gift saying *I love you*—meaning it takes *one* letter to say 'I,' *four* letters to say 'love,' and *three* letters to say 'you.'

When I was in my early teens, my weight began to climb as my body was naturally growing into that of a woman. I was terrified. I thought I was getting fat. My weight was 142. I saw it as my curse speaking, *I hate you*—meaning it takes one letter to say 'I,' four to say 'hate,' and three letters to say 'you.' I was one pound shy of that 143.

My diets began.

I didn't see the weight as a blessing as Mr. Rogers did but rather as a curse. I was fat. I was out of control with food. I didn't love myself, nor my body. My weight was not a gift speaking, "I love you," but rather, "I hate you" because I was worthless, dumb, ugly, and of course, fat.

And so my quest to be thin began. My fear was of not being pretty enough, thin enough, or smart enough. My weight jumped up and down to the highest of a hundred pounds overweight to as low as 129, and everything in between. But that 142 pounds seemed to stick as my set point. No, I didn't see it as a gift at all, but rather as a curse—a curse of self-hate of my body—and hate of the natural progression from girl to woman.

Taking care is the one way to show love are powerful words. Did Mr. Rogers overdo his taking care? No, perhaps not for him, but for me, my overdoing of self-care manifested as obsession with body and with weight. Mr. Rogers, on the other hand, seemed a structured, gentle kind of guy, who followed a daily ritual. A sort of, if "it's not broken, don't fix it" kind of mindset.

I learned after three decades of struggling with my food to build a ritual that worked for me. A ritual of going to bed at the same time and rising at the same time, walking, swimming, or biking daily, eating real foods and avoiding sugar, flour, and wheat, staying away from alcohol and any and all illegal substances. Who knew I had so much in common with Mr. Rogers.

I recognized after years of trial and error, schooling, and working with Weight Watchers of Greater Miami for thirteen years, interacting with the clientele, that some of us had an eating disorder, which needed to be addressed.

I had binge eating disorder, bulimia through *over* exercising, and food addiction.

Eating healthfully, engaging in moderate exercise, and drinking water as my main drink cleared my pimpled face and released my weight, while propelling myself away from sugar, flour, and wheat cleared my addictive craving for junk foods. Today, my weight is stable up and down within a two- to three-pound range, unlike Mr. Rogers who weighed 143, period.

So, as for me, I swing between 138 and 142—ah, here's that number again. Perhaps if I'd been content at the 142 all those years ago, I could have spared myself decades of an eating disorder, self-loathing, and body image distortion. Perhaps.

Alcohol, drugs, poor quality foods, cigarettes all lead to aging poorly. At one time I smoked two packs of menthol cigarettes a day—in the hope of warding off a higher weight. I chose junk foods over alcohol—most of the time—not for health purposes but rather for a calorie bargaining chip.

Drugs. Thank goodness I didn't go down that rabbit hole, but surely I could have, especially cocaine as a weight controller—but my fear of my parents *killing* me kept me from that. And of course, for me, pot was a no no because it would make me eat, or so I thought—also I needed to always be in control—at least where substances were concerned.

Today, no cigarettes, no alcohol, moderate exercise, real food, spiritual nourishment including good books, journaling, and writing are some of the ingredients I employ to live my best life. Also, laughter, smiling, and pure fun are important. Life is a gift we are blessed with; cherishing and respecting it might give us the best opportunity to age gracefully, ward off illnesses—and if we do get sick, maybe we can pass through it quickly.

Life is a good thing. Life means energy. Perhaps the magic elixir is to live for the fulfillment of life — not just for us, but also for others. Perhaps the magic is to wake up with a goal, to rise in the morning with intention — pursuing a life filled with purpose rather than dread of self and body, and looks as we age.

Too many people are defeated by the everyday problems of life — and when the pain is too great, the obsessions kick in to distract. They continue on from struggling with the distraction of not enough money, not skinny enough, or this food will make me feel better — just this once — to *if I were only younger, then....*

Well, guess what? You were young, and perhaps you were obsessing about something else that prevented you from living in the moment. Now, here you are still looking back and wishing. Stop. Step into exactly where you are with love and respect for yourself, and watch the magic begin.

You can permit obstacles to control your mind to the point where they are uppermost and thus become the dominating factors in your thought pattern. Or, you can learn how to toss them from the mind by refusing to become mentally submissive to them, and by channeling spiritual thoughts to rise above obstacles that might have been defeating you. No more.

For sure we face real challenges. I've dealt with many, including a failed first marriage, poverty, skin cancer, obesity, an eating disorder, obsessions and addictions, and much more.

Every human being has a story, and I'm no different. Parts of **My Story** here are adapted from my first three books, as my story hasn't changed — though each book represents a different side of the diet mentality and how it can morph into other manifestations of self-obsession, such as a fixation on aging.

My Start

Very often, the work we choose in order to make a living stems from deep-seated personal experiences. When I was just a small child, I was introduced to the fear of aging when I overheard my dad and mom having an intimate conversation about his upcoming birthday of thirty-something. He was terrified of aging. It was mid-morning and my parents were still in bed as my dad worked late evenings playing the accordion and piano. As an accomplished musician, he had to look and play the part — as young. Even back then, young was in.

I was *that kid* who listened and assessed and processed in my mind what to avoid and what to accept. I was a thinker. At the same time, I had my own issues going on with foods to comfort myself against my fears of the unknown in life. A big bad world lurked out there, and I was scared.

In our house, my parents argued over my mom's weight, money, politics, and a host of other concerns, all of which left me to comfort myself with food. I was also aware that *an end to life awaits us all.* My young mind wasn't ready for such a specific.

I preferred to put my emphasis on sweet, sticky foods, as they were exhilarating, felt good, not to mention tasted good to my newly awakening taste buds. These treats blocked anything negative—like aging, becoming poor or absolutely destitute, or any other such information my immature mind absorbed while most likely understanding the dilemmas out of context, with little logic to sort these questions through.

I evolved as a sneaking, lying, stealing, food-hiding kid afraid of the harsh world out there. This was the 60s, a time filled with violence, riots, wars, and killings. *Let the fears begin…*

My full-blown eating disorder appeared at the tail end of my twelfth year, as I was budding on thirteen. Fortunately, in my late teenage years, I found my way to Weight Watchers and began to lose weight and build confidence, and my mood swings became less volatile.

The original Weight Watchers program back in the mid-1970s, under the guidance of Jean Nidetch, the founder of the organization, followed a "natural" food path adopted from diets used for diabetics in a hospital setting. *I instantly felt relief.* Little did I know at the time that I was sensitive to "processed" foods, which led to binge eating and crazy inner dialogue.

I reached my "healthy" goal weight for the first time at the age of nineteen, and I stayed there and basked in my glory for a whole five minutes. I went on to reach my goal weight three more times, and in my thirties, I finally was able to maintain a hundred-pound loss for ten years by following each new and improved Weight Watchers diet—armed with willpower and a clenched jaw.

With my false sense of success, I went to work for Weight Watchers, thinking I had finally found my ideal solution. But once the novelty of shedding weight had lost its punch, periodic binges, mood swings, terrible fatigue, low self-worth, and low-grade depression again resurfaced, not to mention that the negative inner diet chatter went from a whisper to a roar.

Through diet and exercise, I managed to keep my weight down but not without a terrific battle regarding binge eating and a string of typical food-addict head games. For several weeks, I ate according to the Weight Watchers food plan (which after the 1970s Diabetic Hospital Plan introduced boxed desserts and pasta delights!), then binged on large amounts of sweets and starches over short periods of time while telling myself I deserved to eat—promising to begin my diet the following day.

Out-of-control eating gradually allowed my weight to creep back on, a pound here and a pound there. Before I knew it, thirty-five pounds had found their way back, and I kept none of my old promises to myself. I was petrified that I was headed for a return to daily binges and on my way up to two-hundred-thirty-five pounds

Eventually, I became conscious of a change in my behavior and moods with certain foods, as well as constant fatigue with specific foods. Some foods were so powerful they compelled me to eat enormous amounts, leaving me high, while others simply knocked me out. In either case, I lacked control.

These foods induced anger, anxiety, low self-esteem, and negative inner diet chatter that were all controlling, not to mention terrifying. This discovery was a tremendous breakthrough. My predicament wasn't my fault. I wasn't weak. I had a definite reaction to certain foods.

Still working for Weight Watchers while studying for my Master's degree in mental health, I noticed I wasn't the only one going up and down the rollercoaster of how I ate—so were many Weight Watchers members as well as the staff. I knew they were trying to "diet" the weight off, and like me, were running through the revolving door of Weight Watchers to find the resolution to a weight-loss impasse.

I knew intuitively the answer wasn't just in following the plan, because as wonderful as the program was (and still is), it didn't provide an educated, licensed psychotherapist. A psychotherapist could have walked the members through the *why* they were eating, as well as *what* they were eating, though most wouldn't actually understand the situation if the member had a food sensitivity.

I knew I had to do something about this terrible problem for both myself and for others, so with great trepidation, I left the fold that had initially showed me the way. I was frightened! I felt as if I were leaving

11

the mother's womb as I stumbled off into the dark alone. I took with me little guidance, except knowing that certain foods were causing me to react with extreme highs and lows, and that my spirituality, which I had been brought up to respect, was stagnant because I couldn't see past the next, inevitable, binge.

With awareness, I developed a list of the foods that profoundly increased my cravings, mood swings, and a serious case of fatigue. After I'd worked with hundreds of patients and weight-loss participants and attended a regular twelve-step meeting to fill my spiritual deficit, I found unambiguous answers, and knew I was on the right path at last. I learned, too, that I wasn't alone. The inner chatter was beginning to quiet.

I isolated three specific ingredients that gave me the most egregious side effects: sugar, flour, and wheat. I found when I ate a balanced breakfast, lunch, dinner, and snack, and avoided sugar, flour, and wheat, while at the same time moving toward my spiritual source, my moods stabilized, my weight dropped, and I stopped bingeing. My cravings disappeared, my energy soared, and my depression lifted. And the inner noise began to quiet from a shout to a whisper, to barely audible.

My weight and my relationship with food were a constant struggle for me until I began to understand my chemical reaction to certain foods. After years of trial and error, research, clinical knowledge, weight loss, and stability of weight, I became calm. These days as I've moved into my later years of life, I continue to follow a simple formula, breaking down each meal in terms of structure and commitment rather than eating randomly. I also include daily exercise such as walking or biking along the ocean, and try and live my life as a prayer.

Like you, my life isn't always bliss. But no matter what struggles life presents, I know that binge eating simply is no longer an option for me. Nor are sugars, flour, or wheat on my food list, because I understand that the sleeping giant within (addiction) will wake, and chaos will return with a vengeance if I ingest any of these. I compare my situation to that of a heroin addict who can't have just a smidgeon of heroin; he must abstain completely to stay clean.

When I began to follow these specific guidelines—even when I didn't want to—my negative mind chatter quieted, and for the first time in many years, I could become still and hear the infinite spirit's whispers. I connected to my inner strengths, and a pure understanding emerged in me. I found internal peace, transcendence, and love. Love for myself, others, and the universe evolved inside me.

Not only was I calmer, kinder, and less self-centered, but I began to see a bigger picture. I saw food as real and not real: nature's food and man's food. I chose food of the earth, sea, and air rather than processed and boxed. I turned to my mystical source so that the "noise" in my head ceased, and the addiction flattened. These days, I eat to live rather than live to eat. Healthful foods and a refreshed belief are now my fuel to optimal health, a sustainable weight, and aging gracefully.

And this book, ***Release Your Obsession with Aging: Heal from the Inside Out***, which you hold in your hands (or on your digital reader), brings forth a combination of ways for you to live your best and fullest life without jumping from this fix and that fix to look young. Now, of course, we want to look and feel our best, and if you elect to solicit surgery, creams, and other procedures. Well have at it— nothing wrong with that at all. Only when the obsession is so gripping that you can't live in the now and enjoy the body, mind, and spiritual self do these processes become life sappers.

Start With Self-Care

As quoted at the start of this chapter, "Taking care is the one way to show your love. Take care of you now and that care will pay off for years to come. Create a new way of looking at you—less critical and less jonsing for young, but rather accepting you as you are right now, as being the best you.

Self-care isn't selfish, but rather a loving, kind gesture to yourself. Self-care is not obsessing about this wrinkle, or that wrinkle, but rather about feeding the self-real, whole foods and taking time out for a walk in nature or a swim in the sea.

Self-love is treating yourself with kindness at exactly where you are right now. Yes, right now, not tomorrow or yesterday when you were younger and full of sass and vigor. I don't know about you, but I want to be that cool older lady in her eighties with some swagger, you know, the one who carries herself as if she's got the world by the tail. That one.

Let's break free from obsessive thinking and greet life as it comes, armed and ready because you're practicing self-care and self-love, and employing help from others as you need to, so you can achieve your self-actualization — reaching your personal fulfillment.

Don't fret that the conditions have to be perfect. No such thing as perfect may ever appear. The truth is, you are *still* going to have to take that first step, but not obsessed. If you begin to move in that direction now instead of later, no matter your age, you will be that many steps closer to your ability to handle any aspects of your aging progression this time next year by making healthy, self-love choices.

Congratulations, you've just moved in the self-care direction, investing in yourself by purchasing this book! You're now well on your way. My hope is that what I've written helps you to recognize, deal with, and resolve obsessive aging mentality, understanding where it stems from and how to transition to living in a more spiritually oriented realm.

If my journey lifts and releases you from the pure hell of obsessions, I will, indeed, have accomplished my goal. Now is the time to dial down the obsessive age-defying thinking, and power up your best self. In Chapter 2, we take a peek into your fears revolving around rational and irrational beliefs as you power through maturing.

Personal Inventory Questions

1. We all have a story, so what's yours? You picked up this book because something resonated within you. Are you obsessed with aging? — meaning every day is an invitation for you to critique your progress in the natural cycle of growing older.

2. Self-care and self-love are paramount to aging gracefully so that you can live a full, healthy life. Do you struggle with one or the other, or both?

3. Living a long life is often the goal, but think about increasing the span of healthy life as an even higher goal. Rather than striving for a longer life, how about trying to increase your number of well years — years of complete wellness, or years of life free of dysfunction, symptoms, and health-related problems. This means you'll experience a whole you, body, mind, and spirit. How does that resonate?

4. Self-actualization is what we strive for to become our authentic selves. Have you reached your authentic self at a spiritual level — a want-for-nothing stage? Have you reached your potential, your self-fulfillment?

5. *Taking care is the one way to show love*, are powerful words. Did Mr. Rogers overdo his taking care? As a kid I was stuck on 142 pounds, a number I saw in a negative light that sprang into a close to a three-decade eating disorder. What about you? Do

you have a gripping number that's caused great havoc in your life?

6. I was *that kid* who listened and assessed and processed in my mind what to avoid and what to accept. I was a thinker. What kind of kid were you?

7. Events, politics, world events often mark or define our relationship with food, body, self-image and aging, hence confusing the actual situation with the *feel good feeling* of certain foods. Can you recall situations that frightened you? Did/does food pacify you?

8. Do you find you're sensitive to certain foods? What foods are they, and what happens when you eat them? How do they factor into your relationship with maturing into adulthood and beyond?

9. Do you have a history of your weight fluctuating up and down? When did this start? And did it manifest into a body image, growing-older concern?

10. You can permit obstacles to control your mind to the point where they are uppermost and thus dominate your thought. Or, you can learn how to toss them from the mind by refusing to become mentally submissive to them—and by practicing channeling spiritual thoughts so you can rise above the obstacles supposedly defeating you. What obstacles seem to stand in your way?

Chapter 2

What Are You Afraid Of?

*Life is not measured
by the number of breaths we take,
but by the moments
that take our breath away.
~Origin Unknown*

What are you afraid of? So often we're afraid but don't have a clue about what. And so often the fear is imagined in heights beyond reality. Have you ever noticed that the event behind the fear, once it happens, is nothing like you thought it would be? Why is this so? Could our thoughts be inaccurate?

I loved babies from an early start in life. I always wanted to hold them, nudge my nose into their wrinkly necks and smell that sweet baby smell—a cross between miniature roses and the saltiness of the ocean breeze. The innocence in those eyes and yet the knowing behind them intrigued me. I even loved changing diapers. Everything about babies, I adored — *they took my breath away.* I was in the moment, loving every second — until I learned how we conceive these delightful gems — how we birthed them into the world. Fear gripped!

My eldest sister decided the time had arrived to have the basic 101 talk about sex and babies — she was maybe fourteen at the time, definitely not equipped to deliver the birds and bees conversation, not to mention discuss the birthing process. But for whatever reason, she decided I needed to know. I was *very* young for my age — protected by my private Catholic school upbringing — I hadn't a clue what I was in for.

My version of the process was that you gently pressed your lips against his lips, and voila, you had a baby in you, and then somehow it magically appeared in your arms. You know, the stork flies the little nugget in, and this joyful, gurgling, smiley baby is yours for keeps. Nope. My sister broke the news to me with a diagram she drew, pointing out this and that, accenting the private parts.

I was terrified.

From that moment on, the idea of sex and birthing a baby was not something I wanted any part of. Shortly after, my eating disorder ensued. I don't believe one had anything to do with the other, but gaining weight, sex, and birthing babies — each terrified me. I latched onto fear like a dog with a bone and it weighed on me as a virtual ton of bricks, covering my thoughts for years to come.

I had nothing to base *any* of my fears on, except for what my little brain's visions were telling me. And funny thing was when I did have intimacy, the experience wasn't the way I feared it would be — nor was giving birth to my baby, which I did naturally because I had a fear of needles. Go figure! Yet the weight horror stayed with me for another few decades more.

Where Is The Fear Coming From?

What is fear? Dictionary.com defines fear as a distressing emotion aroused by impending danger, evil, pain, etc., whether the threat is real or imagined. What screams out to me here is "whether the threat is *real or imagined.*" For most of us, being gripped by fear is one of the worst feelings in the world. You can see it in the eyes, voice, and behavior of the person seized with dread — trembling at just the thought of the event, without ever experiencing it.

In my field of practice most of my patients have anxiety. And most of the angst comes from an unknown baseline deep within. The most common fears I hear revealed are apprehension about becoming fat; nervousness concerning adulthood; alarm over sex; fear of people looking at their nose, ears, stomach, etc. — and trepidation over aging. Yep, there it is — fear of aging. And what comes with aging? The idea of aging brings worry over not being mobile, being ill, being alone, losing driving privileges, having money woes—the inevitability of death. And for certain all of these are real possibilities, though they aren't all probabilities.

Think about it. You can be troubled by and fret over imagining not being mobile, or suffering some unforeseen illness—or worse, that you'll be all alone and not have driving privileges, maybe even encounter financial stresses… But what if you start to worry at say age fifty, and *none* of these worries come to fruition, and you pass, let's say, 80 years old. My goodness, thirty quality years were wasted fearing and fussing over something that *might* happen. Or maybe you transition five years later, and lost five good years *living in upset.* No, stay in the now.

Of course, as life happens, you'll have times when you can't exert control over situations that might change the course of your life. Take COVID-19, aka the coronavirus, which recently plagued all of us from sea to sea and land to land—leaving nobody untouched at least on some level. None of us had any power over this, except for how to act or react. For months we stayed hunkered down, except for those of us considered "essential," who went to work.

But most fears aren't founded and aren't caused by a pandemic like the coronavirus. But still we have baselines that are disrupted and stretch far into our adult lives, creating a cascade of fears. Take Minnie, who faced tragic situations during her childhood and into her adulthood. Her baseline, according to her mom, was that of her being a nervous baby; anything loud made her uncomfortable. Minnie came from a vivacious Italian family, a people who are known to excite easily. (I speak from experience, coming from an Italian background, myself.)

At any rate, Minnie had a way of annoying the snot out of her mom, which led her to be given the belt quite often. Minnie never knew when to just sit in silence and let the wave of Mom's wrath pass. No, she'd argue, confront, and even judge—all of which led to a punishment. She was high spirited and curious to know the whats and whys of every situation; hence, she never knew how to simply sit back and be quiet.

Minnie left home in her late teens and set out on her own, connecting with a boyfriend whom she married to begin her adult life, pregnant and young. Minnie was a nervous driver placing one foot on the brake and the other on the gas while driving. One day while driving, she hit the brake too hard on the icy snow and lost control of the car, leading to a terrible car accident.

Minnie wasn't able to walk for months after, requiring lots of treatment, all while taking care of her young toddler, pregnant with the next child, and now immobile. After that cold, dreary winter day, she began to fear driving and only stayed on one-lane roads, still driving with two feet—one on the gas pedal and one on the brake, making for a jerky ride from one destination to another as she stayed under 25 miles an hour, regardless of the speed limit.

Fast-forward, Minnie arrived home by herself but sensed she wasn't alone. Items in her quaint, usually meticulous home were in disarray, and she noted that her underpants and bras were half-hanging out of drawers. She froze, fearing someone was there. She startled when the door burst open, only to find her husband with their then teenage children.

Her husband saw the look on her face and knew something was off. Though nobody else was in the home at that moment, as he slipped out the side door, the news spread on television of a town stalker. After this, someone rummaged through many houses that were home to women and teen girls; soon an arrest was announced, followed by the release of the suspect. Then came the murder of a local victim—all of which left Minnie a nervous person, fearing many things.

Often, when we have fear starting from the baseline, as Minnie experienced while a child, the emotion builds throughout the person's life and can lead to anxiety, depression, and fear of the unknown, such as of the aging process and being alone. Initially, when I began working with Minnie, her reason for contacting me was her incessant fear of aging. But once we unpacked her history, both she and I saw clearly that the fears were based on her anxiety given the experiences she'd had earlier in her life that led to many unwarranted fears.

First, in her earlier years, Minnie feared becoming heavy, so she leaned on one fad diet after the other, and mixed in that she feared driving, and of course loud noise made her antsy. But later the fear of growing old took grip. She feared losing her husband and being left alone and victim to something or someone. The actual death of her husband weighed heavily on her, to the point of her shutting down all outside contact, which led her to psychotherapy.

The Journey

As for death, yes it's inevitable for all of us. And with it can come fear. Maybe you don't realize you even think about dying, but the subject is back there in your mind, whirling as a subconscious fear. Death is another journey in our passages through life. Perhaps making peace with it by leaning on your faith, or attachment to nature as the cycle of life, you can quiet those tones of fears. Or you can worry and feel angst—then transition (pass away) anyway. Hmm, sounds to me as though you'd be wasting a lot of precious life over something that's simply part of our process.

This fear of becoming older, with death pending, can actually start while someone is quite young. Many of my eating disordered patients began the fear at around the age of twelve. I did. I was afraid of adulthood responsibilities, though I was already taking care of myself by the start of my teens. I was afraid of growing up and having to work a "real" job and providing for myself—though I was working my first job at twelve in the pepper fields alongside Mexican migrants.

Of course, back then I was saving money to purchase my horse, Pasha, but I was working, and I was young and earning what I wanted wasn't terribly difficult. In fact, this stint as a worker was a great introduction to adulthood, though early—and yet I feared growing up.

So all my fear of growing up was unfounded as I was already growing up quite young. One minute I was playing with stuffed animals, climbing trees, racing on my bike and playing baseball and kick-the-can with the neighbor kids. And then the next moment, I was living in a fractured family, trying to find wholeness in a chaotic world. You can say my experience was like being thrown in the ocean without a boat, life preserver, or any assistance and expected to swim. Well, swim I did. And so will you...

And falling in love, intimacy, having a child, and all that followed weren't what I imagined. The me in my head feared giving birth and intimacy, but the reality was so far different than the discomfort I pictured in my inner world.

But the reality and my fantasy, I soon learned, were not the same. The day my baby came into the world wasn't what I'd fearfully envisioned. It was good. Giving birth to Benjamin was the most spectacular experience I'd ever had in my life, before and since. The event was miraculous—an out-of-body experience. It was holy, truly phenomenal. I didn't feel a stitch of pain except with the episiotomy—and that involved needles and sewing. And my fear of needles has been at least real and measurable — though I can create a scene in my mind with that too — for sure.

The Unfounded Fear Journey

Most times in life our fears don't emerge as the reality. When I read Jane Fonda's book *My Life So Far* back in 2005, I had no idea what she was talking about, though I thought I did. She spoke of the three arcs, from youth to adulthood to the last stage. Now, as I'm moving closer to my 64th birthday, I get it.

Ms. Fonda felt the milestone of reaching sixty warranted a review of acts one and two where she discovered clear, broad, even universal themes that ran through her life, a coherent arc to her journey. And this arc, I believe, is found in all of our journeys.

Today, as I'm turning the corner into the last act in my life, I read from Ms. Fonda, "It all began as I very intentionally prepared for my sixtieth birthday. Whether we care to admit it or not (and I'm a strong advocate for admitting), sixty marks the start of our third and final act — unless we live into our hundreds. God forbid!"

Well, I'm staring straight into the barrel of my third and final act — and this time is scary yet exciting, all rolled into one. Like Ms. Fonda, I'm hoping my journey, and that of others shared in this book, might provide a road map for you, the reader, as you face the challenges of aging, self-image, and self-love — while you reach toward self-actualization, a true fulfillment.

My hope is that a clear materialization of your authentic self emerges as you discover and connect to your spiritual self.

Interestingly, Ms. Fonda was sixty-two years old and five months when she began writing her book—and I myself was a handful of months past my sixty-third year, when I started *this* book. Ms. Fonda and I share many commonalities with an eating-disorder, exercise-bulimic past. And as with me, her eating disorder and all that came with it followed her throughout much of her first and second act in life.

I have many patients in their third act with the eating disorder still in full bloom clouding their existence as they power through the final years of life. Let's hope this is not you.

So, as this last act unfolds, I'm entering uncharted territory with some fears of the unknown. I don't know, and you don't know, what the coming years may hold, or if they even will be, as we conjure the story in our minds.

One thing for certain, the movie in our minds is never what it is in the flesh, just as the movies you watch on the screen never live up to expectations if you read the book first. Why? Because readers create the visions in their minds according to their experiences; hence, watching the movie created by someone *else's* vision looks and feels different.

So what to do? How do we move through these fears? How do we identify what we're afraid of? Well, we don't. We don't know how our individual stories will play out—but what we do know is we are good right now, in this moment. Live in the now rather than forecasting what you don't know, and you'll find peace. If tomorrow isn't here, and you stay with each breath, you'll breathe your way to a remarkable state of mind. If you remain in the moment, your movie in the mind can't go haywire, creating all these fears to come — as fears to come are in the future not in the now.

So often we run from the fear by fixating on our weight, food, body, money, wrinkles, and all that comes with life's ups and downs.

Do we dye the hair, fix the teeth, and get a nip and tuck here and there? Sure, if that's the actual root of the problem. But often the root of the fear is grander and greater than a snip and tuck. Often, as already noted, what we fear is imagined. Then what? Well, we miss the moments that take our breath away.

Life's Transitions

Most fears begin when people find themselves in life transitions or when situations are out of their comfort zone. And of course fear leads to worry, which leads to the start of "what ifs," and hence, all the scenarios begin to play out in the head. I like to think of this as the story taking residence in our thoughts. Then the story becomes bigger than life, bigger than reality. And when that happens, we can lose control, with our believing each terrifying, imagined thought.

Most of us are not strangers to this mind-crippling, spine-tingling, heart-stomping fear, having experienced the feeling at one time or another. But this is not to say fear is always a bad thing, because many times fear can save our lives. For instance, if you instinctually feel someone is behind you when you're walking, often without pause you turn to look and there someone is. This is a good thing.

Minnie sensed someone had been in her home. And someone was. Becoming afraid was a natural response. We're supposed to have fear, as we've learned in psychology, and react with the instincts of fight or flight.

Fight or flight response, also known as acute stress response, refers to a physiological reaction that occurs in the presence of something frightening— mentally or physically. Interestingly, this response is triggered naturally by the release of hormones that prepare our bodies to deal with what's about to happen, or to flee to safety. I always imagine in this case a bear chasing someone in the woods as the person scurries up the tree to safety.

Today, we aren't in primitive times and most likely don't have bears lurking in the background, but what we do have is traffic, car accidents, loose dogs, financial fears, and losses of many sorts...all of which can trigger a fight or flight response. But we also have an imagination that can trigger the same fight or flight response when nothing has happened—at least not in real time, but rather in the mind's imagination. Minnie's unfounded fears took her in and out of the fight or flight response, which when triggered only by the mind can prove to be unhealthy in the long term.

Fight or flight that comes about with a stress threat, as the bear is chasing or whatever the real-world threat is, serves by protecting us in instances of actual danger. This is a good thing. Fight or flight is not such a good thing when it becomes crippling, and we stress beyond healthy. When we begin to show symptoms of heart issues, headaches, or stomachaches or are paralyzed with such anxiety that we can't carry on simple tasks such as concentrating when reading a book or paper, the fight or flight response is not on our side. Minnie had stomachaches and chest pains due to her crippling fears.

What's Your Personality Type?

Considering the fight or flight response, I'd like to present the personality types and how each might respond in different situations. Often the idea of character and personality are interchanged, but they, in fact, are different, though related. Personality is comprised of inborn traits while character consists of learned behavior. The character may vary with the situation or circumstance or may be purposely changed, based on personality traits.

Personality type refers to the psychological classification of different types of individuals. A type can be introvert or extrovert (discussed in Chapter 9). Personality types most of us are familiar with are Type A and Type B, but as time marched on, some personality charts incorporated different types such as: Type A, B, C, and D, which I find beneficial as these classifications are concise and to the point.

Type A describes the director type who's goal oriented, risk taking, and good under stress, whereas Type B is the socializer, meaning this type is more relationship oriented, outgoing, and enthusiastic. The Type C is the thinker — more detail-oriented, logical, and prepared. And the last type, Type D, is the supporter, who is task oriented, stabilizing, and cautious. All display interesting traits, many of which most of us have some parts of. Type X describes someone having two or more personality types that are equal

When examining the fight or flight response, not uncommonly we find this same kind of stress when a person is a Type A, a highly successful person always on the go, running here and there, which generally puts the body in an automatic alarm state — not always such a beneficial thing. As you can see, fight or flight serves us best when the bear is chasing us, versus when we chase success and don't allow ourselves a breather.

The Type A tends to have this need to be in charge and in control of their environment and their lives. This type is hard driving and ambitious, with perfectionist thinking. They also often tend to work independently and set their own schedules. In addition, they tend to be workaholics, putting in whatever time and effort they need to accomplish their goal, paying less attention to relaxing...smelling the roses kind of thing. With Type A, it's push push push...which leads to exhaustion and often spikes the fight or flight response.

31

The Type B personality is very outgoing, energetic, and fast paced. They love to be around other people and enjoy being the center of attention. They are likeable and tend to be relationship builders. They love to talk about themselves and have a great need to be liked. Most important to this discussion of aging is that the Type B doesn't want to appear unattractive or unsuccessful—making sure their appearance is impeccable while they make certain to give the impression of being VERY successful, whether true or not. This can turn into a fight or flight response as well.

The Type C personality is a very detail-oriented fellow who likes to be involved in events that are controlled and stable. They are most interested in accuracy, rationality, and logic. They avoid those who can't seem to control their emotions. They also avoid those full of hype. The C type tends to be quite controlling—both of themselves and others. They don't like situations to get out of hand—nor do they express their emotions. And of course we can't control that which comes with the aging journey, which can cause the fight or flight response.

And then we have the D personality type, who takes the slower, easier pace toward life in general. They do seek security and longevity in whatever their interests are—glad to work in a repetitive pattern, which allows them to become quite skilled at the task at hand. This type requires a secure, stable environment to feel okay. As long as the environment is secure, the stable calm remains.

Regardless of which type you are, you can find a way to navigate through the ups and downs of life as you journey through. The theme behind all of my writings is our ability to heal from the inside out. When we are in such distress, long term, the upset is quite harmful, causing many debilitating symptoms such as anxiety and depression and feelings of sadness or emptiness, all which can lead to accelerated aging.

Additionally, constant distress can lead to extreme irritability over small or insignificant things. Anxiety and restlessness may lead to difficulty concentrating or staying in the moment. The result here can be a loss of interest in activities we once loved, like cooking, cycling, reading, etc.

This heightened state can lead to an adrenaline rush, which is quite addictive— necessary from time to time to keep us pursuing and creating. But when we overdo the adrenaline spike, this is not a good thing physically. Adrenaline is a hormone secreted by the adrenal glands, especially in conditions of stress, increasing rates of blood circulation, breathing, and carbohydrate metabolism, and preparing muscles for exertions.

Adrenaline is normally produced by both the adrenal glands and a small number of neurons in the medulla oblongata, where it acts as a neurotransmitter involved in regulating visceral functions (i.e., respiration). Adrenaline is also known as epinephrine, which is a hormone and medication.

What happens to the body in this response, physically? Well, your face will either flush or pale, your eyes will show dilated pupils; most likely you'll be trembling, and for sure, you'll experience a rapid heartbeat and accelerated breathing. This set of reactions is terrifying, not to mention harmful to your body, mind, and spirit. And our goal is always to work on physical, mental, emotional, and spiritual health throughout our lives, regardless of age. The power to heal is yours.

The fear of becoming sick—or the big C, as my patient Sadie described cancer, can be quite frightening—especially if it comes into fruition. Though Sadie greeted her diagnosis with open arms from start to end, the illness emerged with a vengeance and took her life in a mere six weeks. That's real. But the entire time rather than measuring life by the number of breaths she took, she measured the moments by the times when life took her breath away, literally and figuratively.

Sadie lived her best life and greeted her transition with the same openness as she had accepted many challenges she had faced. Witnessing this patient greet life as it handed her end-sentence was priceless for those around her. She taught the biggest lesson of all—to embrace the now—not what might be tomorrow and not what she should have done in the past.

Surely Sadie made peace with her regrets and mistakes, but that came long before she was struck by cancer. She'd already learned to live in her moment, watching the events unfold and take her breath away rather than counting each breath she took. She accepted her cancer, not that it defined her, but rather as something in the hands of her higher source.

Sadie understood she was following the will of a source greater than she was—a timetable that wasn't hers to will. I'm not saying that she didn't want to heal or that she didn't wish for a longer life, because she did. But she also wasn't without a hope that she would encounter another realm to her journey. She found her peace and went with it.

This experience I witnessed Sadie go through took *my* breath away because I learned that life is about the here and the now—not tomorrow. And I saw that Sadie had memories of fabulous moments in life and was grateful. She was ready to greet the other side and see her loved ones. She had a strong spiritual composition, and that carried her from start to end.

Of course, facing death is a frightening experience when you're not at peace with yourself, your higher connection—whatever that will be—and those around you, whether nature or family and friends. Fears come in all shades; some, as you will note, are real, and others are fabricated in the mind. What happens then when illness comes? What is conjured in the mind? As we grow older, from birth to transition, most often some illnesses will pass our way. How can we manage in a positive light? Turn to Chapter 3 and learn how we can deal when illness happens.

Personal Inventory Questions

1. What are you afraid of? So often we are afraid but don't have a clue about what. And so often the fear is imagined in heights beyond reality. Can you pinpoint your fear(s)?

2. Have you ever noticed that the event behind the fear, once it happens, is nothing as you thought it would be? Why is this so?

3. What is fear? Dictionary.com defines fear as a distressing emotion aroused by impending danger, evil, pain, etc., whether the threat is real or imagined. What screams out is the idea of whether the threat is *real or imagined*. Was your most gripping fear real, or imagined? And how did it impact your life journey?

4. The most common fears I hear are fear of getting fat; fear of adulthood; fear of sex; fear of people looking at their nose, ears, stomach—and fear of aging. Do you fear aging? What parts of the process are most concerning for you?

5. Minnie had some tragic situations occur during her childhood as well as in her adulthood. Her baseline, according to her mom, was that of her being a nervous baby. Anything loud made her uncomfortable. Minnie came from a vivacious, Italian family, known to excite easily. What type of family do you come from? Has it affected your fear barometer?

6. This fear of growing older, with death pending, can start quite young. Many of my eating disordered patients began the fear at age twelve. I

did, too. At what age can you mark the start of your fears? How has it impacted your daily life?

7. Most fears begin when people find themselves in life transitions or when situations are out of their comfort zone. And of course, fear leads to worry, which leads to the start of "what ifs"; hence, all the scenarios begin to play out in the head. What are your "what ifs" and how do they mess with your balance of life?

8. Sadie greeted her cancer with open arms, grateful for her life experiences. Can you relate to her openness? What, if anything, would you do differently?

9. Type A is the director type who's goal oriented, risk taking, and good under stress, whereas Type B is the socializer, meaning this type is more relationship oriented, outgoing, and enthusiastic. The Type C is the thinker—more detail-oriented, logical, and prepared. And the last type, Type D, is the supporter, who is task oriented, stabilizing, and cautious. What type are you and how has it impacted your fight or flight response?

10. When I read Jane Fonda's book *My Life So Far* back in 2005, I had no idea what she was talking about, though I thought I did. She spoke of the three arcs, from youth to adulthood to the last stage. Now, as I'm moving closer to my 64th birthday, I get it. What arc are you in? Do you see your life as arcs, seasons, or chapters? Or do you see life as one straight line of experiences?

Chapter 3

When Illness Happens

The future belongs to those who
believe in the beauty of their dreams.
~Eleanor Roosevelt

How can one believe in the beauty of their dreams
when illness strikes? Especially since the onset of
COVID-19, coronavirus — this shook the foundation of
most of us and our institutions. What will the future
entail? A pandemic such as this can leave many
wobbly about their dreams. Doesn't the future
become dim at best?

The thought of any illness looming can be
crippling for us, especially when such a devastating
disease is widespread. But suppose our dreams can
carry us through the dark days, lending hope to

possibilities. Suppose mere thoughts can turn our direction positive or negative, depending on what thoughts we feed our expectations.

The mind is powerful, and our anticipation can change the course of our outcomes. If we believe an illness, any illness, is going to kidnap our dreams, then it well may. But remember, not all illnesses inevitably lead to doom and gloom. In fact, often an illness can be an awakening. How many times have you heard someone say they are thankful for the illness because it turned their life around — and maybe even connected them to a higher source they once neglected?

An influential, fearless writer, Howard Rankin, PhD, author of *I Think Therefore I Am Wrong: A Guide to Bias, Political Correctness, Fake News and the Future of Mankind* offers suggestions and tools as to how we can, as individuals, improve emotional control — a critical component for more critical and objective thinking.

Dr. Rankin teaches how advertising and media train our brains. This is not farfetched when we think about how "young is in and old is out" — a message touted non-stop, day in and day out. It's a message we hear without cessation from every avenue we can imagine — a training of the brain, so to speak.

In fact, case in point, on my twitter feed one of my twitter friends posted a question, "If you could wave a magic wand, what would you change in your life right now?" I pondered for a second and posted,

"Nothing." But as I perused the other responses, I saw many wanting back their youth.

One answer in particular grabbed my attention. This woman wrote: "My age. I would change my age. I would be young so it wasn't embarrassing for me to ask for help from others who are mostly younger and definitely more intelligent — including here. Swallowing being the adult who solicits support and is helped by *kids* is hard."

I swear, I'm not making this stuff up. There, glaring right in front of me was that to be young is the gold piece. Is it? Okay, so maybe the being ill part isn't so hot, but guess what, youth falls sick too.

We all, at every age, may have an illness to contend with. But today, illnesses that are a possibility are jumping right at us from the advertisement venue. Yes, they remind us about the lurking illnesses and remedies that are to come. Remedies like this medicine and that medicine will give you relief, or comfort, or maybe even a cure.

And what about the mental health medicines blaring from the television, radio, billboards, and magazine ads? If you listen, really listen, you can almost convince yourself you have the very mental illness the pill is promising to erase or at least give relief from. Yep, another training of the brain that for sure we need a pill for this or for that so we can be "normal"...*whatever that is.*

One commercial after another spouts that we can erase this or tuck that or remove that sag, wrinkle, or impurity, which I discuss in Chapter 4, concerning surgeries. Each advertisement trains our brains to believe we aren't good enough, smart enough, thin enough, or young enough *as we are,* or that we're sick and need medicines for our illnesses.

The messages insinuate that what we have going, in the now, is awful and we need a snip or two to make us beautiful — i.e. acceptable. Or that a pill will correct the thoughts in the head — and, of course, at times it will and is necessary, but for sure that's not the norm.

In spite of the media efforts, another rumbling is going on that says we can change the course of our lives through our thoughts. Perhaps we can think ourselves well.

Think Yourself Well

Not long ago I was listening to a powerful podcast, entitled "How Not to Think About...Cancer," launched by Dr. Rankin on January 8th, 2020. The premise of the show was how the right mindset can beat cancer.

For the record, I'm a podcast junky, and once I'm hooked I listen to every interview or podcast release, and this series was no exception. In fact, I was honored to be a guest on the podcast myself back on March 2nd, 2020: "How Not to Think about...the Chatter in Your Head Concerning Your Weight and Body Image"

—a takeoff on my second book: *Release Your Obsession with Diet Chatter: Heal from the Inside Out.*

Long before I was ever considered to speak on this podcast, I was listening to one of the programs that really stayed with me. The guest, Johann Ilgenfritz, had been given six to twelve months to live when cancer infiltrated in his body. Johann, a photographic journalist in 2011, only forty-six years old, believed that he had other ways to conceptualize his situation. He began to question conventional views and the suppositions often tied with the diagnosis of cancer — or any disease for that matter.

Prior to the cancer diagnosis, Mr. Ilgenfritz had a heart attack, then shortly after learned he had cancer, which first was treated with conventional medicines. But when the cancer returned with a vengeance, he changed his thoughts — which altered the course of his life.

Within three years, Johann was cancer free, which led him to founding UKHealthRadio — one of my current favorite radio stations, as it's filled with a plethora of health and wellness experts from all over, providing varied perspectives and opening the mind to options of all sorts.

Johann Ilgenfritz revealed how he changed his mind set as he moved into a health-packed regimen using natural remedies. I'm not suggesting readers use natural over conventional treatments, but I am suggesting that the power of the mind can make a difference in how we handle situations in our lives whatever approach we take.

In the second book in my obsession series, *Release Your Obsession with Mind Chatter: Heal from the Inside*

Out, I speak to the power of the mind to change thoughts and reactions. The process is a simple but powerful one wherein your thoughts pass from your conscious mind to your subconscious, which in turn influences your actions in accordance with these thoughts.

So, for instance, if my conscious thought is *I am a weak person*, that thought will pass to my subconscious mind, which in turn influences my action in alignment with this thought. In other words, I will behave as though I'm weak.

As noted, Mr. Ilgenfritz did go the route of conventional medical treatment, but then shortly after, learned he had terminal cancer and was given six to twelve months to live. He painted a vivid picture for his podcast audience as he remembered the first time he was diagnosed and how the news filled him with terror, putting him in a daze. But this was **not** his reaction with the return of the cancer, which led to the thought *this is not going to happen*. He then had a three-year-old son and was determined not to miss the boy's milestones.

Johann's conscious thought was *this is not going to happen*, and that thought passed to his subconscious mind, which in turn influenced his action in accordance with his thought.

This type of news can affect people differently. Remember earlier in Chapter 2 Sadie referred to cancer as "the big C," where she greeted her news with acceptance and open arms, from start to end. Her conscious thought was *this is happening*, and that thought passed to her subconscious mind, which in turn influenced her action in accordance with her thought. Unlike Johann, she received, claimed, and owned her cancer and called it cancer, whereas he didn't even like to have the *word* cancer in his vocabulary or thoughts.

As noted, Sadie's cancer came on with a vengeance, as did Johann's, but in Sadie's case, her life ended in six weeks. Most important to note, Sadie was ready to exit. She felt she had completed what she had to. Her children were grown, and she was tired. Did she give up? No. She simply had a different mindset than Johann did. She was ready to end this chapter.

Sadie lived her best life and greeted her transition with the same openness with which she had gone through her life. Those witnessing Sadie received her end-sentence as a tragic one, but she did not. She taught the rest of us the biggest lesson of all — to embrace the now — not looking to what might happen tomorrow and not what she should have done in the past. She felt fulfilled — she had achieved self-actualization, and was ready for her journey to the unknown.

So here we have two stories of a terminal illness, one person changing and "believing" his conscious thought of *it's not happening*, while the other owning the diagnosis and accepting that *it's happening*. As stated, Sadie made peace with her regrets and mistakes, but that came *long before* she developed cancer.

Sadie had already learned to live in her moment and watch events unfold, taking her breath away (in a positive sense), rather than counting each breath she took. She accepted her cancer, not that it defined her, but rather allowing it to be in the hands of her higher source. And she felt her time served here was complete.

Illness will come for all of us, and we have options as to how we receive it. We have choices regarding taking either conventional, or alternative measures in treatment—and whether to work with the mind in one direction or another. That's the point—we have alternatives. One pick isn't necessarily better than the other, but rather, what counts is how you greet the decision.

You might be thinking, *Wait. Hold your horses. Are you saying someone who passed away from a heart attack chose that heart attack?* No, maybe not chose the heart attack, but believed they had a bad heart and perhaps chose to ignore it and continue the same lifestyle that promoted the bad heart in the first place.

The power of the thought is huge—and can change the course of your life. And what you choose to do also changes the outcome. How we work through our illnesses is part of working through the aging process with grace, dignity, and acceptance. Both stories above are positive stories from the actors in their own points of view. For us as readers, we may ponder how the woman's death could be a constructive outcome—but it was. Sadie was ready and went with it.

A Knee Can Let You Down...Or Not

Illnesses can be physical and they can be mental, both of which can be crippling. A man I knew, Jared, comes to mind; he had learned he might be a candidate for knee surgery. Jared suffered from a type of mental illness consisting of high anxiety, coupled with irrational beliefs. He was on a host of anti-anxiety, anti-depression, and sleep-aid medications. He experienced panic attacks, which turned into panic disorder.

Jared created a scenario in his mind that he would be crippled, in a wheelchair, and that nobody would take care of him. Jared had plenty of funds, and he was physically strong, yet went through anxiety to the point he couldn't sleep without waking with a panic attack several times a night. He *believed* his life was over, that he was old. He accepted that when you're old you'd need knee and hip surgery because relatives of his had needed these surgeries.

Jared was so convinced his time on this earth was coming to a close that he went as far as settling his accounts, financial as well as social media, so his wife could take care of the finances and wrap up "his story" online when he was gone. For sure, he was putting the cart before the horse in his negative thinking.

And when this fellow Jared said, *"when he was gone,"* he meant dead—out of this world gone. Jared already had himself dead and buried when the doctor only suggested *maybe*—and a weak maybe—that he'd need knee surgery—not a knee replacement, mind you, but rather a meniscus repair.

My understanding is that a meniscus tear means a torn meniscus, which is one of the most common knee injuries. Each of our knees has two C-shaped pieces of cartilage that act like cushions between our shinbones and our thighbones (menisci). A torn meniscus causes pain, swelling, and stiffness. Knee arthroscopy is often used to treat a meniscus tear. Depending on the tear, however, some tears heal by themselves.

In Jared's case, his story took on a life of its own when the doctor said he *might* need surgery at some point. But the very same doctor also offered many options to avoid treatment with an intrusive operation.

The doctor believed the patient could build the muscle around the knee and avoid an intrusive procedure altogether. But the doctor's belief is not the healing potion; the patient himself needed to believe—to have that knowing to create a different outcome. Our thoughts are powerful, perhaps even more powerful than our action, as it's the starting place for all things to sprout.

Please note I'm NOT saying we can cure ourselves with our thoughts, but what I'm saying is we can create an illness when we have none, and that in some situations, our beliefs can turn around the outcome of a diagnosed illness. For certain, going to the doctor and getting a work-up is in order, but beyond that, you do have the opportunity to work with your thoughts and how they can interrupt your progress or help immeasurably.

Thank goodness I was able to work with Jared at the onset of his "story" and begin to use cognitive behavioral therapy and hypnosis to redirect his subconscious mind, which feeds the conscious mind.

Cognitive behavioral therapy, also known as CBT, is a form of psychological treatment that has been demonstrated to be effective for a range of problems including anxiety disorders, depression, and eating disorders. This style of therapy approaches faulty and/or irrational thinking, learned patterns of unhelpful behavior, and poor coping skills. The goal is to change the thinking patterns and assist the patient with relaxation therapies and strategies to utilize while not in session.

And the hypnosis or hypnotherapy brings the patient into a trance-like state in which that person has heightened focus and concentration. I use hypnotherapy in tandem with CBT to assist in quieting the mind and redirecting the faulty thinking to rational thinking. The goal is to gently move the patient into focused attention while reducing peripheral awareness, thus enhancing the patient's capacity to respond to suggestions. We build a list together that is used for suggestion.

Jared turned off his irrational thinking and turned on resolutions and solutions. He did, in fact, go to physical therapy with the intent of working the muscles around the affected area. To his delight, now, he is not only living on, but he is climbing stairs and cycling along the beach daily.

Belinda, on the other hand, a blonde-haired, blue-eyed diver was not so lucky and did need the knee arthroscopy to treat the meniscus tear in her right knee. She was open and ready for the procedure, believing it would be quick, followed by physical therapy, and then she'd be as good as new. And she was. She's diving and teaching yoga, and power-walking with her Great Dane. Belinda's mindset was one of positive beliefs she'd be up and about in no time. Both Belinda and Jared were in their early sixties.

So, as you see, we can create scenarios of all sorts with our minds. And along with that, we can see through a positive lens, no matter the choice made. Your choice might not couple up with another's, and it doesn't have to. We each have our own peace within — our own personal narrative.

Health Options

Many health options are available to redirect our future health, and one is the food we eat. The old adage, *you are what you eat,* is a powerful statement that still holds true today — on the *inside and the outside* of your body. Food feeds thoughts as well as the body — internally and externally. Eating properly, meaning real, non-processed foods that heal, can assist the efficiency of your digestive system, organs, mental prowess, and energy.

Sadie, who accepted her death, had a long history of obesity, eating processed foods, and living a sedentary life, all of which may have contributed to her early passing at the age of 62.

The fellow who refused to accept his diagnosis, Johann, to the point he didn't even keep the word *cancer* in his vocabulary, turned to whole, organic plant foods and fared well. Jared, the man with the possible knee surgery was thin and looked fit, but predominantly ate processed carbohydrate foods — and healed nonetheless. And Belinda ate only whole, non-processed foods. She had surgery, then healed quickly. All four people's stories were rooted in four different human situations with different outcomes.

Now you might be thinking how could food play such a role in our health? It does. It plays a huge role — maybe as big as our thoughts. Choose real food such as plant foods grown in the ground or foods off a tree or perhaps harvested from the floor of the sea, and you are off to a good start.

What is generally known these days is that food affects you internally, as already suggested, and your outward appearance as well, including your weight, visual signs of aging, and the condition of your skin. In addition, food can affect our thoughts via our mood along with our concentration, as you will see when I delve deeper into the possibility of slowing the aging process with foods in the chapter on food, mood, and wrinkles.

Some aging foods include high sodium snacks, not to mention alcohol and manufactured types of harmful fats, all aging foods that can lead to illnesses. Although caffeine is touted as being good for you, too much is never a good thing. Caffeine acts as a diuretic, drying out the skin, giving one an older appearance.

We need to drink fluids throughout the day in order to hydrate because our bodies lose water through our breath, sweating, and digestion. And shockingly, many do not like water because it is tasteless. But our body and blood are largely made of water and so we need to be drinking water. Other animals instinctively do, and at one time we humans did, too — that was until other flavored drinks came into the picture, making plain water not so desirable.

I know of a patient, Mara, who had a strong aversion to water and never drank it. She loved coffee, and though coffee is made up with water, water is only a part of the mix. Mara also ate an unvarying diet, consisting mostly of carbohydrates such as oatmeal, apples, Ritz crackers, and cream cheese...while drinking loads of coffee.

Today, she has osteoporosis, meaning porous bones with many small holes, so that liquid or gases can pass through. This is a disease in which the density and quality of bone are seriously reduced. As bones become more permeable, one is at risk of fracture — and Mara is turning the corner and entering her nineties.

Yes, Mara's had a long and prosperous life, filled with a strong faith and family connections. All good. But she stoops over with a bulge in her back and lives in chronic pain. She never exercised, as she thought it a waste of productive time, and barely took time to eat, since she was a workaholic through and through. Her lifestyle has now caught up to her, and perhaps it didn't have to.

Mara, on a positive note, never *ever* went out in the sun, so her skin is porcelain without a wrinkle in sight, and yet she uses no fancy creams nor has ever engaged in surgeries of any kind. But imagine where she might be in her life today if she had drunk the miracle substance known as water and stepped back from having so much coffee.

It's not news that with a poor diet, smoking cigarettes, consuming loads of caffeine, alcohol, and/or sugar, you *will* appear older than your actual age, not to mention irritate your inner organs. Sadie, who passed away in six weeks after her diagnosis, had a tendency to eat deli ham, bacon, sausage, and hot dogs as her main staples, along with white bread and cakes with thick icing from the local grocery store—all addictive and destructive foods.

The man with the knee issues, Jared, tended to eat slightly better but leaned more toward skipping meals and carbohydrate loading, avoiding protein altogether. And he always saw the glass half empty; not believing anything good could come out of his challenges in life. But he worked on himself with psychotherapy, hypnotherapy, and healthful eating, and turned himself around. He is on his way to a productive last chapter in his life.

And then there's Johann, who changed the course of his life through staying away from all processed foods, and eating organic, so that he is still here today. He was blessed to see all of his children grow and soar in life. He took his illness to a constructive outcome by creating an entire radio station promoting positive health.

Belinda, who was innately optimistic and active, ate whole, natural foods and believed in the best in all situations. Though she had plenty of hurdles in life, such as the early death of her husband and having no children when she desperately wanted babies — and being at one time drug addicted — she powered through. She overcame life's adversities. Today Belinda is a happy, productive woman teaching yoga and traveling the world, giving power talks about healing from drug addiction — a disease, for sure.

I'm not saying a healthy mind and healthy foods are the only answer to all of our ills, but I'm merely offering a comparison of several situations of mental and physical illness, all with very different outcomes for different reasons.

And what about surgeries? It's possible that sometime in your life as you go through the aging process, you'll need a surgery. Let's see what surgeries these might be in Chapter 4.

Personal Inventory Questions

1. "The future belongs to those who believe in the beauty of their dreams," said Eleanor Roosevelt. What do you think about that? Does the future

belong to you when you have an illness looming over you? Examine your thoughts on this and see what bubbles up.

2. The mind is powerful, and our thoughts can change the course of the outcome. If we believe the illness is going to kidnap our dreams, then it will. Not all illnesses lead to doom and gloom. What thoughts did you have as you read these lines? Did it anger you? In what way?

3. What about Howard Rankin, PhD, author of *I Think Therefore I Am Wrong: A Guide to Bias, Political Correctness, Fake News and the Future of Mankind*, who suggested, "Advertising and media train your brain." Do you think this is so? Perhaps you can recall an advertisement or something in the media that trained your brain. How did it impact your thinking — and behavior?

4. What about your social media feed? Have you ever read something that made you ponder about your life? I know I did when I read on my twitter feed the question, "If you could wave a magic wand, what would you change in your life right now?" What have you read?

5. At the start of the chapter, I presented two cancer cases with two very different outcomes. The first was that of Johann Ilgenfritz, who refused to *believe* the cancer would take his life in six to twelve months, and the second was Sadie, who was told her cancer was terminal and to get her papers in order. Do you think our minds are so

powerful that they can determine life or death? Have you ever experienced anything like this?

6. And then we have Jared, who really made quite the story in his mind about his knee. His tale was totally inaccurate, yet he believed it to be true. Often with illnesses such as anxiety, our minds can become quite crafty and make up situations that are not so. Have you done this? Or are you more like Belinda and power through a situation expecting a positive outcome?

7. Food is an integral part of our health options; leading us possibly to very long and healthy lives and/or possibly help to not only offset an illness but also maybe help you through it. What kinds of foods do you tend to eat?

8. Now you might be thinking how could food, a simple thing such as nourishment, be so important? How could food play a role in our health? It does. It plays a huge role—maybe as big as our thought. What do you think? Could our thinking go wayward based on how we eat?

9. And what about water? Are you one to drink water? What is the impact for you with or without proper fluid intake?

10. This lovely woman in her nineties had porcelain skin from not going in the sun, yet also had osteoporosis, due to her diet and lack of water intake. Is having a youthful-looking face most important to you?

Chapter 4

Surgeries Call You

What lies behind us,
and what lies before us
are tiny matters compared
to what lies within us.
~Ralph Waldo Emerson

There are surgeries and there are surgeries. One type you don't voluntarily sign up for, and the other you do. The surgeries such as heart, thyroid, removal of cancer, and a host of others, are a choice, but often a necessity, if you want to live. So though you do volunteer, you do so because if you don't, the consequences may be grave. But the truly voluntary, the elective surgeries, are another ball of wax.

This chapter focuses on cosmetic surgeries, the voluntary surgery that engages in improving our appearance. You know, the ones that aren't actually necessary but rather a "luxury," or perhaps a bow to vanity. These operations spring from the obsession over an aspect of how someone looks that makes the person feel less than, maybe undesirable — from his or her perspective, of course.

And since I live near Miami, a noted hub of plastic surgeries, elective procedures become more of a topic of discussion for my patients with eating disorders, which always hinge on associated areas of body image and appearance, considerations lurking in the background for those with food issues.

I'm not suggesting cosmetic surgery is a terrible thing, but I am suggesting that we can be beautiful exactly as we are. I'm also suggesting that sometimes the obsession over chasing youth can drive our desperation to a point of us proceeding without caution, especially if we're promised amazing results.

Miami is a major center as well for troubled cosmetic surgery clinics, ballyhooed by discount prices and social media advertising that targets obsessed, desperate persons yearning for the promised youth, no matter the actual physical cost.

In *USA Today* and *Naples Daily News*, on December 5th 2019, an article appeared entitled, "This Business Helped Transform Miami into a National Plastic Surgery Destination: Eight Women Died," written by Michael Sallah and Maria Perez. The article features a Miami plastic surgery empire that attracted patients from across the U.S. with the promise of inexpensive procedures and life-changing results.

Using social media channels such as Facebook, YouTube, and Instagram and marketing to a population desperate for the promises of youth at an affordable price, and with payment plans in place, bad things began to happen.

Bad things, such as eight women dying within a short span of time. The cosmetic surgery facility in question had undergone multiple name changes over the years, but the same doctor, Dr. Ismael Labrador, was present in all the business operations...along with his wife, an attorney whose law firm defended the many accusations of malpractice.

Dr. Labrador's clinic, despite the name changes, was among more than a dozen high-volume clinics that transformed Florida into a national destination for plastic surgery. Some of the surgeries included the Brazilian butt lift, tummy tucks, and eyebrow transformations, along with many other procedures.

Some cosmetic surgery may well be necessary, such as after a disabling incident like a burn from a fire or a catastrophic accident that left the patient disfigured. A terrible tragedy of some sort can cause scars, or a person may be born with a disfigurement requiring correction, or some physical situation may be crippling the person's productive life. Those persons facing such impairments deserve the help plastic surgeons can and do provide. This is *not* the type of cosmetic surgery I'm referring to.

In fact, any cosmetic or improvement type surgery is fantastic and a good thing. However, the surgeries that become *obsessive* and crippling due to the monkey chatter in someone's mind are the ones we want to eradicate, because they are simply not healthy.

The surgeries I'm referring to are the types provided by clinics that are owned by investors and driven by social media marketing offering discount prices that attract thousands of patents each year across the country. We can be vulnerable to such marketing when the promises sound so grand that they will transform our lives to a sort we only dreamed of having. Does that sound familiar? Similar to the "lose the 20 pounds in 20 days" diet that will give you the body you always dreamed of, these surgical offerings send out pretty much an identical message, but the product is generally more dangerous—and more alluring.

I can't tell you how many times I've said to my husband that I'd like a mini facelift or an eyelift, or something to take away my "tired" look. And every time he pulls me close to him, saying, "I love you just the way you are. Why would you want to mess with your beautiful face? Leave it alone." I'm thankful his response isn't something like, "Yes, Lisa, you should get a little tuck or nip—that'd be good."

The negative chatter whispers in our heads that we need to change this or that to look amazing. We all get caught up in this from time to time—and I'm no different. Thank goodness my husband doesn't support my negative chatter, because if he did, I'd maybe fall down the rabbit hole so many are pulled into. Does the inner self drive the outer self or the outer self-drive the inner self? A question to ponder perhaps.

What Lies Within

What lies behind us, and what lies before us truly are tiny matters compared to what lies within us. We could take that saying a step farther and look at our youth, which lies behind us, or our future aged self that we are growing into — but neither being as important as what we carry within us.

Our inner being is the be-all from start to end. I mentioned in the opening of this book that my good friend Susan once said to me she felt exactly the same inside her mind at her present age as she did at her earlier ages. I was only in my thirties, and she was about to complete her fifties. Fast forward to the now, I'm in my sixties and share her view. My thoughts and beliefs and morals are all intact from back then to now. The mechanical body's inner and outer workings are what is changing.

And Susan and I are not the only ones who feel young in our minds; so does Jennifer Lopez...and even Oprah. I was listening to Oprah's *Super Soul Conversations* (on OWN) while walking with Gracie the other day, and to Oprah's guest, Jennifer Lopez, in the March 4th show entitled "Oprah and Jennifer Lopez: Your Life in Focus" from Oprah's 2020 Vision Tour in Las Angeles in front of a live audience. The crowd was pumped and roaring ready for the conversation Oprah and Jennifer Lopez were about to have.

At some point in the discussion, Jennifer Lopez talked about how she'd turned 50 years old the prior summer. Oprah said to her, "I read somewhere...you don't feel like you're aging, you just feel like yourself. The number doesn't even mean anything."

And Jennifer said, "I honestly feel the same way I did when I was 28 and put out my first record." Then she went on to add, "I think it's a mindset, just continuing to realize I'm still growing. And as long as I'm growing, I still have somewhere to go. That there's more to journey, and not just because I turned fifty, my life is over." And when she said, "It's not over—we're just at halftime," of course the crowd (of mostly women) shrieked with uncontrollable shouts of joy.

We should all have that *We're just at halftime attitude.* Of course if you watched the last Super Bowl, you'd know why the audience broke into applause and laughter and screeched with joy, because fifty-year-old Jennifer Lopez and Shakira, a forty-three-year-old knockout worked a dynamic duo that delivered the South Florida vibe together with the Latin ambiance.

If you remember the game played on Sunday, February 2nd at Hard Rock Stadium in Miami Gardens, Florida, the San Francisco 49ers played the Kansas City Chiefs. The Super Bowl was thought to be a great game, with Miami written all over it,

61

putting the crowd in an excited, heightened state. The two sizzling women performed moves most of us never could imagine attempting in our twenties let alone our forties and fifties—proving age is just a number.

Hearing Oprah in her upper sixties and Jennifer Lopez now fifty speak to aging the way I believe aging is was refreshing. It's a mindset. And though we may be at an advanced age according to society, we harbor the same type of thoughts as in our youth and know we are the same person that lies within us.

Yet we see around us a mad rush to look young. The necessity for youth is front and center to many in our society—especially women. I've made no secret of the fact that this book revolves around a body image perspective. I'm an eating disorder specialist and most of my patients struggle to shape their bodies as they wish, and in time, as they age, their faces become the target of obsession, along with the aging process itself. Aging steps up to the hyper focus, pushing the eating disorder to a second-place position...and this progression includes men, mind you.

Men want to feel young and look young too, but may not be as desperate as women—or at least the need presents a little differently. Men's top priorities seem to be to display muscles and to perform in the bedroom, while women are focused on presentation rather than performance. Both aspects of personal insecurities can be equally crippling.

One of my sons went to five stores *during the coronavirus pandemic*, looking for exercise equipment because his gym closed. He was frantically trying to put together the same schedule he was used to performing at the gym for the last twenty-five years. He was desperate enough, forgetting about the deadly virus, to meander through not one but FIVE stores, only to find shelf after shelf of gym paraphernalia gone. Then he went to the internet.

He found nothing.

Why? Because hundreds or thousands of men (and women) undertaking the same quest to work out other than at the gym, were scattering to find machines. In fact, one of my patients ordered a Boflex fitness machine promising an at-home workout in preparation for the closing of the gyms.

And I witnessed a fellow, I'd guess in his upper fifties, working out by the beach with a makeshift gym he pulled out of his bag. He pumped away with an ocean breeze and view to go along with it.

This searching to recreate a gym can, of course, be a very good thing, showing the need to take care of our health during trying times. This is a positive way to live our best lives in our best bodies, following a natural, holistic path. All good.

Changing Ideals Of Modern Society

I remember when I was working on my Master's, then doctorate, in my thirties and early forties respectively, one reading assignment from my biological psychology course imprinted in my mind forever. This bit was from the book *Biological*

Psychology: An Introduction to Behavioral, Cognitive, and Clinical Neuroscience, right in Chapter 13.

The chapter began with a story of a California woman in 1998 who was sentenced to a two-year probation because her daughter, at age 13, weighing 680 pounds, had died of complications from obesity. You can bet I was hooked and read on, as my own eating disorder was running rampant at the age of 13. And due to the amount of binge eating I did, I could easily have been at a high weight like this teen. And here I was working on my Master's degree all these years later, coming from the overweight teen still struggling to calm the blazing-hot food addiction.

The story went on to discuss all the diets this teen had been on with no luck. I could relate. The child was so ashamed of her weight, she held herself hostage in her home, refusing to attend school. Again, I could relate. I skipped school all the time when I was in grade school as well as high school. Though I wasn't enormous — yet — I feared I was headed that way. In time, I made my way to one hundred pounds heavier than my five-foot-six frame could handle.

Although this teen didn't wish to be obese, she was. She tried diet after diet to no avail. I believe she had food addiction, something I suffered from, and a named compulsion nobody knew about back then. And even today, many close their eyes to such a serious disease. I was heartbroken reading this teen's story because the uncontrollable disease of food addiction is not always seen as real. The old adage, just eat less and exercise more, seems to take front and center, missing the point completely.

In a related tragedy, still in Chapter 13, the story went on about male wrestlers in college trying to lose weight quickly before a tournament. The young men followed the traditional route of subjecting themselves to high heat so they could sweat and lose fluid...but they went too far and died of heart failure. They died! They died because they wanted to wrestle with a certain weight class and needed to lose weight quickly. Guess what? This still goes on today—as do cases similar to that of the young girl who died from obesity.

Anything To Stay Young

Okay you ask, what does this have to do with cosmetic surgery. Nothing. Except, we will do anything to look a certain way—including accepting the risk of death. Remember Joan Rivers? Joan Rivers, a well-known comedic celebrity, died on September 4th, 2014, at the age of eighty-one, days after she stopped breathing when undergoing a routine endoscopy at Yorkville Endoscopy in New York City.

The allegation was that doctors at the clinic mishandled Ms. Rivers' procedure by performing a laryngoscopy on her vocal cords without consent rather than the prescribed endoscopy. The autopsy revealed that Rivers' "official cause of death" was brain damage from lack of oxygen. A lawsuit undertaken by her daughter, Melissa, ensued over the clinic's commitment to provide quality and compassionate health care services—both sides agreeing to a settlement.

The story is tragic because prior to the incident Ms. Rivers joked regarding her plethora of plastic surgeries. Death is no laughing matter for sure, but the irony was that she passed away from a simple procedure when she'd had a series of plastic surgeries in the course of her adult life. The public and media view seemed to be that she was addicted to plastic surgery and went too far trying to maintain her youth.

If you ask anyone in their upper fifties and beyond how Joan Rivers passed away, you're sure to hear she died from a mishap during a cosmetic procedure—though she didn't. But the public can't think of Ms. Rivers without tying her to plastic surgery.

Joan Rivers admitted to having had lots of plastic surgery, including a facelift neck lift, and eyelid surgery—and seemed to make no apologies or excuses. She was born Joan Alexandra Molinsky, but was known professionally as Joan Rivers. She was an American comedian, actress, writer, producer, and television host.

When I think of Joan Rivers I think about her often-controversial comedic persona. She knocked herself, just as much as others knocked her, but she also had a knack for picking apart celebrities and politicians. Though thinking of Joan Rivers without thinking about her sharp tongue and wit is hard, it's also hard not thinking about her as the queen of plastic surgeries.

In several interviews she stated she had been overweight throughout her childhood and adolescence, and that this had a profound impact on her body image, which she struggled with throughout her life. And that's the point I'm trying to make — that often body image, weight, and all that comes with it morphs into an obsession with looks and aging.

When young, the focus is on body weight and looks, and when old, the struggle involves chasing youth and looking young. In that same book *Biological Psychology: An Introduction to Behavioral, Cognitive, and Clinical Neuroscience*, right in Chapter 13 was a section on the two common eating disorders, bulimia and anorexia. And next to the section were two photos, one of an almost anorexic-looking movie star, actress Lara Flynn Boyle, dressed in a gown for a gala event, and the other of Helena Fourment, the Flemish painter Paul Ruben's wife, in *Helena Fourment as Aphrodite* (circa 1630), both of which exemplified ideal feminine forms of their respective eras.

In today's world, Helena Fourment would be considered morbidly obese. Yes, morbidly obese. But back then, she was considered a real beauty to emulate — different eras for sure. Critics often suggest that our modern weight-conscious notions of female beauty are responsible for many cases of anorexia nervosa and bulimia. I'd like to take the theory a step farther and say that in our modern body-centered society of today, not only must you look thin and waiflike, but also you must look young.

From my observation, more and more teens and young adults are considering plastic surgery due to peer pressure and the bombardment of messages that old is bad and young is good. Add to that list the many different reasons plastic surgery is becoming the rage today from social media pressure, to television advertisements, billboards, peer pressure, and the influence of social circles. The feeling of not belonging or being good enough seems to fuel the desire as well.

What I see in my work is a belief that if the person can look a certain way, then all their wishes will come into fruition. They'll find the right partner, money will become plentiful, and they'll be accepted and fit into the social set of their dreams *if only* they present as young, thin, and beautiful—or handsome and strong.

I recall one woman nearing her eighties believing reaching a certain weight and looking younger would bring her happiness. She elected to have an eyelift, tummy tuck, facelift, and breast reduction, a nose job (rhinoplasty) to change the shape of her nose—not to improve its function—along with a breast lift. Though she already looked lovely, she wasn't happy. Why? She wasn't looking within but rather behind and forward. She still was suffering within not feeling good enough.

The tragedy was this woman, nearing her eighties, had spent years and years thinking she was homely. She spent thousands upon thousands of dollars trying to look young, as the parents who raised her didn't believe she'd amount to anything because she wasn't beautiful, according to their standards. They were distant and cold, rarely if ever hugging or complimenting her. She believed their opinion that she wasn't going to be good enough. They regularly reminded her that she was homely. She believed them.

Many people don't see or believe in their inner or outer beauty, based on degrading messages from earlier years—most if not all not even true. Imagine if you were told how beautiful you were inside and out from the start—not in a egoic kind of way but rather in a spiritual, *God's child* kind of way—what a difference that could make. Beauty, they say, is in the eye of the beholder. I ask, who is this beholder, the one looking at you or you looking at yourself?

The beholder is an observer, someone who gains awareness of things through the senses, especially sight. If beauty is in the eye of the beholder, then the person who is observing gets to decide what is beautiful. I say we are all beautiful, and beautiful in every moment.

What's scary is if "beauty is in the eye of the beholder" means beauty doesn't exist on its own, but is created by observers. The beholder may take in different aspects of the other, but I say beauty should be in the eye of the persons reflecting on themselves. Why do we need an outsider opinion to decide our beauty?

I always remember the actress Jennifer Grey, who played opposite Patrick Swayze in *Dirty Dancing* back in 1987, and who all but disappeared after that film. Many criticized her for her nose. Then a dramatic "nose job from hell" led to the star and her burgeoning career taking a very different path.

"I went into the operating room a celebrity and came out anonymous," Jennifer Grey told *The Mirror* in 2012. She went on to say, "It was the nose job from hell. I'll always be this once-famous actress nobody recognizes because of a nose job." How tragic, as she was stunning as she was. Imagine if the striking Barbara Streisand had changed her nose. Would she have disappeared into the ether as well?

Often our beauty is our authentic look—not a "plastic" look.

Why Plastic Surgery

In the *Canadian Journal of Plastic Surgery* article entitled "Factors That Motivate People to Undergo Cosmetic Surgery" investigators revealed many interesting insights as to why people elect to turn to cosmetic surgery. And though the research focused on women, many men elect to have surgery as well.

For this study, a sample of 204 British participants completed a questionnaire assessing their reasons for surgery and measured self-esteem, life satisfaction, self-rated physical attractiveness, religiousness, and media consumption. What was fascinating was the attitude regarding surgery revealed by the participants.

Two factors emerged as to who is likely to undergo surgery. Females with low self-esteem, low life satisfaction, low self-rated attractiveness, and few religious beliefs, who were also heavy television watchers, reported a greater likelihood of undergoing cosmetic surgery.

The article points out that cosmetic surgery is concerned with the "maintenance, restoration or enhancement of one's physical appearance through surgical and medical techniques." The American Society for Aesthetic Plastic Surgery reported an increase of 446 percent in cosmetic procedures since 1997 — and 8 percent in 2007, with a 17 percent increase in men undertaking cosmetic surgery. And since the numbers have risen exponentially, almost the new norm might be to have a nip, tuck, or change to some part of the body. This was especially true prior to the pandemic because of technological advances in cosmetic surgeries, which made them safer and less invasive, with faster recovery, and of course lowered costs of the procedures. While this has been enticing to many, we can only wonder if the rise in these surgeries will hold up after the COVID-19 diminishes in impact.

However, what motivates people remains constant in being low self-esteem, media exposure promoting a miraculous change, and of course the promise that an "improvement" will be seen regarding the surgical candidate's *flaw*, an upgrade that will lift the person's confidence. What is most interesting is the religious impact on those who may struggle between wanting to look a certain way versus accepting their God-given gift of natural beauty, which is the backbone of this book. The ideal here is to be less concerned with physical appearance—and to realize that true beauty lies within, as the individual's spirit. The idea that what lies behind us and what lies before us are tiny matters compared to what lies within us speaks volumes.

As we move on from surgeries possibly calling us because we want to change this or that for a newer and more version of improved ourselves, we shall have to peek at the question of weight and muscle. Now you may be asking, "What's muscle got to do with it?" I say plenty...turn the pages to Chapter 5, and you'll soon learn the connection between body weight and muscle tone as it relates to the obsession with aging and how to release it.

Personal Inventory Questions

1. "What lies behind us and what lies before us are tiny matters compared to what lies within us" speaks volumes. If Ralph Waldo Emerson were sitting across the table from you, what would you want to ask him about this quote? What parts of this quote speak most to you?
2. What are your thoughts regarding surgeries in general? When was your last surgery, and how did it affect you? Would you do it again?
3. So often our minds are young while our bodies are aging. Are you the same person inside that you were during your younger years? What changed?

4. When did you first notice your fixation on your body and aging? Were you like the young girl in high school who was overweight and stayed home from school? Or what about the young athletes sweating to make weight for their sport? Do your earlier years feed into your quest to be young?

5. Working with the addiction, eating disorder, anxiety, and depression population every day opened my eyes to how many are so focused on the aging process. Are you focused on the aging process? Did you suffer from an addiction or an eating disorder of some sort? What about anxiety or depression? Do you find any of these disorders also triggered a focus on the aging process?

6. With social media channels such as Facebook, YouTube, and Instagram marketing to a population desperate for the promises of youth at an affordable price, with payment plans in place, bad things began to happen in Miami. Have you ever been lured by a marketing scheme, wanting to do some type of cosmetic surgery? If so, looking back, was the decision good for you? Did you find the youth you were seeking?

7. Oprah said to Jennifer Lopez, "I read...you don't feel as if you're aging. You just feel like yourself. The number doesn't even mean anything." Then Jennifer said, "I honestly feel the same way I did when I was 28 and put out my first record." Do you believe you can feel in your later years the same as in your early years? Is it a mindset? How old do you feel in your mind?

8. Many people don't see or believe in their inner or outer beauty, based on degrading messages from earlier years—most, if not all, not even true. Imagine if you were told how beautiful you were inside and out from the start—not in a egoic kind of way but rather in a spiritual, *God's child* kind of way, what a difference that could make. What messages did you hear and how has it impacted your view of yourself?

9. If you ask anyone in his or her upper fifties and beyond how Joan Rivers passed away, you're sure to hear she died from a mishap during a cosmetic procedure—and she didn't. Do you think about plastic surgery and Joan Rivers in the same thought? What impact has she had on you and your belief about cosmetic surgery?

10. In research reported in the *Canadian Journal of Plastic Surgery*, two factors emerged as to who is likely to undergo surgery. Females with low self-esteem, low life satisfaction, low self-rated attractiveness and few religious beliefs, who were heavy television watchers, reported a greater likelihood of undergoing cosmetic surgery. Do you fit in any of these categories? And if so, do you struggle between your religious convictions and the decision to change a body part? Does one collide with the other, and if so, how does this conflict with who you see yourself as?

Chapter 5

What's Muscle Got to Do with It?

Twenty years from now,
you will be more disappointed
by the things you didn't do
than by the ones you did.
So throw off the bowlines.
Sail away from the safe harbor.
Catch the trade winds in your sail.
Explore. Dream.
~Mark Twain

As you look back on your life so far, do you wish you had lived differently? What would you change? Often I hear, "If only I knew then what I know now, my life today would be so different." Does this hold true for you? What didn't you do that you wish you had? Do you wish you had been thinner, or that you had written that book you thought about — or do you wish you had been stronger, more fit, then, and now?

We always have the opportunity to work on a dream, whatever that might be. As we age, we might begin to feel the dream slipping away. Or the body is changing, and we have no control. Both men and women go through changes, similar and not so similar, but frequently weight plays a role in the changes — gains and losses.

With the gains and losses, too, often we experience a skeletal muscle change. And I've heard said that skeletal muscle is the fountain of youth.

For women, changes are precipitated by the decline in estrogen, which generally drops when women reach menopause. This downward slope affects everything from our moods to our midsections, which can explain the melancholy disposition to the flabby midriff, to skeletal muscle change.

And men also go through changes as they age, often leading to their being less active. Yet consistent exercise (activity of all sorts) preserves lean muscle mass and strength, which commonly declines in sedentary aging adults.

In Harvard Health Publishing's article, "Preserve Your Muscle Mass," age-related muscle loss is reported as a natural part of aging. But the Harvard Medical School publication says that doesn't mean you're helpless to stop the decline. While men will typically lose as much as 3 percent to 5 percent of muscle per decade, women lose muscle at a slower rate; however, the muscle cells of men are more responsive to a protein meal than are women's.

Despite the decline in muscle mass as we age, known as sarcopenia, the news isn't all dismal. Putting forth consistent effort to increase muscle can slow down the depletion. The loss for men is partly attributable to a natural decline in testosterone, a hormone that stimulates protein syntheses and muscle growth, and for women the hormone estrogen, which declines when women reach menopause, is a component in the loss of muscle mass.

And with that muscle loss comes greater weakness and less mobility, and sadly an increase in our risk of falls and fractures. That lean muscle mass and strength commonly decline in sedentary aging adults doesn't have to be our personal outcome. We can stop that loss; the choice is within our control. Regular exercise preserves muscle mass.

How do we build muscle mass? Lift weights. No, not lifting weights like Arnold Schwarzenegger, the Austrian-American actor, filmmaker, businessman, author, and former governor of California (2003-2011), and most importantly to this point, a professional bodybuilder. No, we lift weights to our personal ability for our health only, not to compete with a full-blown weightlifter.

The news here is good. The Harvard article states that just because we lose muscle mass doesn't mean it's gone forever. Dr. Thomas W. Storer, director of the exercise physiology and physical function lab at Harvard-affiliated Brigham and Women's Hospital says, "Older [adults] can indeed increase muscle mass lost as a consequence of aging."

Dr. Storer goes on to say, "It takes work, dedication, and a plan, but it is never too late to rebuild muscle and maintain it." And this applies to women as well. Though weightlifting in the past was synonymous with men lifting, this is no longer the case. Women are lifting too, and the benefits are exponential.

Though hormones complicate the process, the benefits of weightlifting are relevant during every life stage—for men AND for women. A plethora of studies also support a mind-muscle connection, indicating moderately depressed people who strength-trained two or more days per week reported seeing their symptoms subside. This reduction in that blue disposition is shown as also true with other types of aerobic exercise, such as walking, cycling, and so on.

Miraculous Change

Many years back, Sara, a boisterous Italian-American, sprinted into my office full of vim and vinegar, and the wisdom only years of experience can bring. At the time she was ending a relationship with a man twenty years younger than she. The relationship with Andy had been toxic, leaving her anxious and irritable. She was afraid to leave him because he threatened to harm her two young sons.

Sara had a bad case of asthma that had begun in her early forties triggered by cheap perfume, bleach, smoke, ammonia, and a whiff of a bad cigar. She was in a bad way. We worked on various means for her to build confidence and move on with her life. After years of abuse, Sara did leave Andy, and voila, the asthma disappeared. No longer did she end up in the emergency room at least once a month, and she began to blossom.

Sara turned to real foods, walked daily, fit in prayer and meditation, and found her way back to her Catholic faith, attending Mass and building friendships. She was amazed at the power of her mind. When she made the decision to turn her life around by changing her thoughts and behavior and reconnecting to her higher source, the miracles began to take hold.

Once Sara's moods stabilized, she released weight, built muscle tone, and found an amazing job working as a private-duty nurse. I didn't see her anymore; that was, until nine years later.

Sara's asthma returned worse than ever. A condition that she used to be able to control, once again became uncontrollable. The thought of going to the emergency room terrified her because of the cost for what insurance didn't cover. Again, money was short, and times were changing for the worse.

Tears tumbled from Sara's eyes, which startled her, as she wasn't one to cry. She was about to lose her job of 10 years caring for Dan, an elderly man she grew to love like family, but now at ninety-nine he was rapidly declining and about to be transported to a nursing home. The family would no longer need her services.

Sara slipped into a dark hole, feeling useless and fearful of what was to come. She was about to go through another major change and feared the unknown. Sara had been walking daily and eating fresh fruits and vegetables, lean proteins, and quality fats with fabulous starches, all of which had nourished her body. She had dropped her excess weight, and on her five-foot-three frame, she was looking and feeling *mighty hot* as she said. But since she'd stopped walking and had begun to eat fast foods again, the weight was climbing, her muscle tone deteriorating, and her asthma had come on with a vengeance.

Sara was lonely and filled with fear. She wished she could have an emotional-assist dog, but with her asthma and allergies, she believed this wasn't an option. The depression worsened, and her energy dipped. On top of this, she admitted she now would become anxious, accompanied by a fast heart rate that made her feel as if her heart was going to burst out of her chest.

What did the body weight and muscle tone have to do with this? Everything. Our physical health affects our mental health, as noted at the start of this chapter, and with Sara the impact was no different. She blurted out at one point, "It's my body! It's not behaving for me. I'm becoming more and more tired as the days pass. I have no energy to walk, and my legs hurt. I'm an old woman, and I'm falling apart."

Sara was 75 years old.

Though Sara was quite naturally stunning and had been quite fit, this new turn of events—losing her job and yet another relationship—she returned to old behaviors of yesteryear. I suggested to Sara that she go to the doctor, have her heart checked along with her breathing, since, as she expressed, she wasn't getting enough oxygen.

Sara was NOT a complainer. This was big, and she didn't feel right. She claimed that the cause was gaining her weight back. I say the fear of losing her job together with the company of Dan, the elder she cared for and was attached to, all contributed to her binge eating, which she engaged in to block her depressed mood, leaving her mentally, physically, and spiritually broken.

Sara slipped back into some old destructive behaviors. She again moved away from her strong Catholic faith, stopped going to church or hanging out with her friends for fellowship. Sara severed her relationship with her long-time girlfriends and broke up with her boyfriend of the prior eight years. Though he wasn't abusive like her previous boyfriend, he hadn't added quality to her life but made her feel bad about herself.

Starting over, looking for a partner at this stage of her life, was devastating and challenging to Sara, not to mention the difficulty of looking for a new job. She felt her current stage was a repeat of the breakup with her prior boyfriend when she and I first met all those years ago.

Sara questioned her future, as many do as they turn the corner and launch into the last act of their lives. Before returning to therapy, Sara had sunk so low that she considered looking into an assisted living situation for herself. This surprised me, as Sara was normally vibrant and free spirited, having the mind and attitude of a young thirty-something.

Sara, as noted, was not a complainer, nor was she one to give up. She was a trooper who had learned to see the glass half full and saw sunshine when the clouds hung low, and laughter when most would call for sadness. She knew how to find her joy, purpose, and value. I reminded her of this. We discussed at length her strengths, and in time, I saw a hint of sparkle return to her golden-brown eyes.

I reminded Sara that this situation wasn't the same as the one when I first met her. She had grown leaps and bounds over the years and endured many trials and tribulations, but sometimes when we have too many challenges at one time, our burdens create the perfect storm. Sara had suffered from bronchitis nine years before, which prompted her to quit smoking, said to be more difficult than quitting heroin. She found ways to control her asthma. In addition, Sara was a heavy drinker back then, so drinking promoted smoking and vice versa. Over time, she had made great strides.

Again, psychotherapy coupled together with daily plans, allowed Sara to grow in her recovery. She had been raised in a non-practicing Catholic family and yearned for that something to cling to. She learned healthy coping behaviors, such as returning to unprocessed foods, exercising, praying, meditating, writing, and using proven techniques to calm the asthma. She now thought she was past breathing issues and weight issues, and that she wouldn't have sore hips and legs if she walked daily.

I asked Sara if she was more disappointed by the things she didn't do when she was fifty versus the things she did. At seventy-five years old, she was turning the corner to a new chapter in her life. She pondered a bit before she answered. Sara now had short, pitch-black hair with the same poignant golden-brown eyes and still maintained her spitfire personality to go with it. She lived like nobody else in her youth—and still does today, at least from my view.

But I wondered from her view what this Italian, Catholic girl with a strong faith would say.

After a long pause, Sara said she wouldn't change a thing with the exception of moving closer to her faith earlier in her life, and she wouldn't abandon her faith every time circumstances became tough to deal with. As she had grown stronger in her earlier recovery, she had built a strong spiritual foundation, but as life happened, she went through a desert spell.

Plug In Spiritually

In time, Sara began to rekindle her faith in God and in herself. She worked through not having a job by taking special interest in her health, and looked fabulous, more content than usual. She *believed* the right job would find her—and it did. Sara lived frugally, depending on her savings to see her through. She stopped eating fast foods and returned to fresh fruits and vegetables lean meats, and good sources of fats and carbohydrates. She melted down to the size she felt best at—once again releasing fifty pounds, looking lean and toned.

When Sara had lost sight of her abilities, she sank to a low as the weight piled on. She felt fat and frumpy, as she frequently would say. When she became heavier, the weight took a toll on her physically, mentally, and spiritually.

Sara had gained a tremendous amount of weight on her small frame, contributing to her rapid "aging," or so the case seemed to her. But once she changed her attitude and plugged back into her spiritual connection, ate healthfully, and exercised, she became the hot, spunky girl I always knew her to be.

All her aches and pains disappeared. She laughed, saying, "I'm still an old person, and some of those pains remain, but now I can breathe, and I feel fabulous." All her major symptoms disappeared. And then soon a job came to fruition—an amazing job with an elderly man who needed an assistant to move in. The job paid triple the salary of the last position, and the pluses consisted of paid vacation, Sundays off, evenings off, and a bonus of $20,000, to begin.

When I was at the start of my recovery from bulimia and food addiction, I was disconnected from my spiritual self. Yes, I had my traditional religion, Catholicism, to fall back on, but that wasn't really feeding my soul. My adherence to church and rituals was giving me rules and guidelines that I'd learned long ago as a child — and for sure I cherish these, but I needed a natural plug-in to my higher source.

In my early days of recovery, I learned about many ways to embrace spirituality. I first found my way through Food Addicts Anonymous, a twelve-step program that was a lifesaver as it provided the spiritual nourishment I craved. At that time I had lost nearly a hundred pounds from my five-foot-six frame, but the weight was slowly creeping back on because I was dieting rather than recovering.

The aging process isn't that much different. In fact, it's not different at all. I was doing an online therapy session during the heat of the COVID-19 pandemic, and a patient, we'll call her Annika, leaned into the screen from her end saying, "Look, look, LOOK at this!!" with total disdain. She was a sixty-three-year-old, gorgeous woman of Swedish descent.

I leaned in, squinted my eyes, and looked as close as I could get my face to the screen, inching in closer and closer, trying to see what this handsome woman was fretting over. Try as I might, I saw nothing but peaches and cream skin, clear cobalt-blue eyes, a perfect button nose, and full lips.

What?

What was she so horrified by? This was a Meryl Streep or a Nicole Kidman type with stunning looks and skin to go with it. She lived in a plush condominium overlooking the ocean with a view to stop anyone in their tracks with awe. In other words, Annika lived a spectacular life in South Beach, Florida where the beach bustled with activity nearly all hours of the day and night.

What was missing? Well, from Annika perspective, she claimed she didn't know how to plug into her spiritual side. Sadly, that's not an ability I believe can be taught; spirituality has to be acquired through the journey. She begged for it, but didn't lean into it the way Sara did early in life, then lost it, but through her hardships found it again.

Some folks have to reach rock bottom to find their way to their higher self, while others seem to grasp it early and hang onto it throughout their lives, and still others never find it at all. Every journey is unique to its traveler.

At my lowest point in life, when I was in my twelve-step group, I not only connected with a community of people who shared their innermost selves with each other, we bared our souls. We were raw and exposed in our pain, totally broken, only to build strong in our recovery.

Annika viewed life from a victim's lens, connecting, owning, and believing in her health issues, some of which were real, and many that were created in her mind. She researched online every illness, hiccup, spot, wrinkle, or blemish that she thought she found or imagined she had, then owned it, and went with it, though all were self-diagnosed.

So here we sat, separated by distance and connected by a screen, where Annika was reeling in *her* real pain, though much imagined. But, whether real or ~~not~~, the pain hurt and hurt bad for her. She leaned in even closer, saying, "Look at these god-awful freckles, gray hair, and saggy skin. I'm getting fatter and fatter. I have no muscle tone, and I'm uglier and uglier being shut in."

I honestly only saw pure beauty in Annika. Of course I could have told her until the cows came home that she was naturally blessed with incredible beauty, and she wouldn't have believed me.

Like many of us, Annika wasn't able to get her monthly maintenance for her hair, so her gray was coming in, and her soft auburn curls were growing long, not to mention her perfectly manicured and pedicured nails were growing out, looking in great need of attention as we were closing in on week seven of virus confinement.

Annika was not spiritual, religious, or connected to anything but her fixation on staying and chasing being young. She was jonsing for her salon, massages, and other pampering. She was more about having Botox when it was allowed again, blocking out people dying, becoming sick, or being placed on ventilators. This was what the obsession with aging will do to a soul. The fixation grips you and makes this quest your total journey in life. You can't think about others, but only about your inner and outer struggles with yourself.

For many of us who found our way to a twelve-step program, or some type of self-help for our addictions and obsessions, we began to grasp our problem was more than a brain disorder. I always find science seeing addiction as solely a brain disorder interesting when spirituality is an essential part of recovery.

Annika never found her way to a twelve-step program for her age addiction, as I don't believe a specific one exists. I've always wondered what would happen if every individual took a twelve-step course of some sort, whether they'd find their path to a spiritual self. My recovery opened up my child wonder — and I became that bright-eyed person full of love, purity, joy, and hope.

Of course that childlike state isn't constant. I'm human and can lose my calm in some situations just like the next person, but for the most part I feel bathed in God's love, and experience the spirit within. And for sure not everyone attending a twelve-step group finds their bliss of love, purity, joy, and hope, but many do. Again, this journey with spirituality appears at its own time and according to its own pace...

So what does weight and muscle have to do with aging? Everything. You see Sara embracing the love and Annika blocking it. Two lovely women, with different views, and two different outcomes — one finds peace and tranquility, while the other stays hyper focused on her body. Sara tapped into her spiritual recovery and a spiritual community whereas

Annika remained an isolator, depending only on herself and her looks. And sadly, our looks and our own company are never enough.

Interestingly, I've known Annika on and off for over two decades as I've known Sara. I'm reminded of the quote I started this chapter with: "Twenty years from now, you will be more disappointed by the things you didn't do, than by the ones you did. So throw off the blow lines. Sail away from the safe harbor. Catch the trade winds in your sails. Explore. Dream."

I remember saying something of that sort to Annika many years back. "You don't want to be in your sixties and still be stuck in the same situation. Sometimes you have to take the plunge and move outside of yourself, though that may be uncomfortable, in order to find your bliss." Well, she didn't. And now she's still singing the same tune she sang back then, and to be sure she may well continue the song in her eighties too.

Don't let this be you...sail away from the safe harbor, catch the trade winds in your sail so that you can explore and dream—no matter your age, as time waits for no one.

Chapter 6 plugs into the Fear of Death, which can come early in life or later in life, or for some, not at all. We are all going to transition at some point, but how we embrace the journey makes all the difference.

Personal Inventory Questions

1. "Twenty years from now you will be more disappointed by the things you didn't do than by the ones you did. So throw off the bowlines. Sail away from the safe harbor. Catch the trade winds in your sails. Explore. Dream." ~Mark Twain... What do you wish you'd done twenty years ago that you didn't do? Can you do that now? How would your life change if this wish came to fruition?

2. We always have the opportunity to work on a dream, whatever that might be. As we age, we might begin to feel the control over our body slipping away. For women, our aging results from the decline in estrogen, this generally diminishes when women reach menopause. For you, if you are a woman, how did the decline in estrogen impact you? After reading this chapter what can you do now to make a difference?

3. And men don't get away without a loss of muscle, either. But consistent exercise preserves lean muscle mass and strength, which commonly decline in sedentary aging adults. And I've heard that skeletal muscle is the fountain of youth. Have you, if you're a man, found a way to regain your muscles? If not, what would it be like for you to feel strong and fit? How would that change your life today?

4. For both men and women, consistently exercising preserves lean muscle mass and strength, which commonly decline in sedentary aging adults. This

is wonderful news! What exercise can you bring into your life right now? And if you already have a workout plan in motion, what can you do to build off of it to make you even more fit and feeling youthful?

5. Many years back, Sara, a boisterous Italian-American, sprinted into my office full of vim and vinegar, and the wisdom only years of experience can bring. She was going through much heartbreak at a later stage of her life. What losses come to mind for you on your aging journey? How did they impact you?

6. Sara began to eat real foods, walk daily, worked in prayer and meditation, and found her way back to her Catholic faith, attending Mass and building friendships. She was amazed at the power of the mind. Do you think changing your thoughts can change your life?

7. Sara had bronchitis nine years before, which prompted her to quit smoking. She thought she was past breathing issues and weight issues, and that she wouldn't have sore hips and legs if she walked daily. Do you believe we go back to previous issues without realizing it?

8. Once Sara changed her attitude and plugged back into her spiritual connection and ate healthfully and exercised, she became the hot, spunky girl she was always known to be. Are you the hot and spunky girl you were meant to be? Or if you're a man, are you the *GQ* hunk you once were?

9. Do you find spirituality plays a key role in your staying youthful? Annika didn't have a spiritual base to turn to. With that in mind, do you think that lack directed the course of her life? What spiritual connections do you have, and how have they helped you maintain your youthful self?

10. Do you find you return to previous mistakes over and over in life at different times? Do you find those mistakes lead to overeating and packing the weight back on that you once thought you rid yourself of for life? Does weight make you feel old?

Chapter 6

The Fear of Death

There are only two ways to live your life.
One is as though nothing is a miracle.
The other as if everything is.
~Albert Einstein

Most people don't think about death or the fear of dying with intensity until it is peering around the corner, either from the loss of a loved one or an illness we ourselves are battling. But when death becomes a reality, the light bulb flashes with the possibility it may not be so far away, after all.

Several months back, the television news blared out some rumblings about a virus in China. Most of us barely listened, thinking China and the few other places the virus had invaded were super-far away.

The talk about this virus continued and became more and more of a topic of discussion, to the point that even the impeachment of President Trump went by the wayside, as did the campaigns for the new Democratic nominee while this pandemic went viral. What was this mysterious virus? Who could catch it? And what was it called?

This mysterious virus came by many names but we seemed to settle with the novel coronavirus being known as COVID-19. Talk soon became non-stop chatter as COVID-19 moved in on all parts of the world, particularly China and Italy early on, and then New York City—the disease in all these places screaming out of control. Although origin sites have been used in the past to identify new viruses, people now realized naming a disease after a region would be seen as denigrating.

The frightening truth was that everyone appeared vulnerable to contracting this highly contagious disease, including young and old, black and white, and everyone in between—but the elderly and those with compromised health appeared to be most vulnerable. Death was on the rise in regions affected, and was the topic daily. How many had this virus? How many had already died from this virus? And talk focused on when would this end; to considerations of how could we prevent contracting it?

We were told we might protect ourselves and help prevent transmitting the virus to others if we:
- Wore a face covering when in public.

- Washed our hands regularly for 20 seconds with soap and water or alcohol-based hand sanitizer.
- Covered our noses and mouths with a disposable tissue or flexed elbow when we coughed or sneezed.
- Avoided close contact (one meter or three feet— which soon changed to six feet) with all people rather than only those people who were unwell, as detecting who had the virus and who didn't was impossible.
- Stayed home and self-isolated from others in the household if we felt unwell.
- Didn't touch our eyes, noses, or mouths if our hands weren't clean.

The name bounced around at the start, but it seems COVID-19 is where it settled. CO and VI come from coronavirus, and the D stands for disease. The 19 stands for 2019, the year the first cases were detected.

This virus seemed to be far away and not much of a concern from all the way over here in South Florida. But, as predicted, it made its way here in record time, and the entire world was soon in a pandemic fury, deeply worried about what would happen next.

Death a Reality

One anxious patient, Roslyn, feared this was the end of the world — that we were all going to die. She was scared. The entirety of our previous and current psychotherapy work seemed to slip out into the ether, because…well, because we were all going to die, anyway. Prior to the virus pandemic, Roslyn's concern was all about aging and cosmetic surgery. But this soon changed.

Now the emphasis for Roslyn became death and dying. Gripped with fear, she no longer would leave her home. We moved our sessions from in-office to video sessions. I used a secure format that worked from almost all devices, allowing my patients easy connection with me if they chose not to come to the office. This connection delivered simple access, free group video calls, screen sharing, and instant messaging, with a secure interface.

The sessions with Roslyn will be forever imprinted in my mind as she always had her screen tilted somehow, leaving me either the view of one big bluish-gray eye filling the screen or only her nose spanning from top to bottom. Or sometimes the screen was tilted completely upside down, leaving me with the sight of her exquisite wood-plank cedar ceiling, the knotted beams stretching the length of the room.

Not every patient saw the virus the same way; some were nonchalant, like Mike, a strong construction-worker fellow, who refused to believe this virus was *that* serious. Mike thought the COVID was being blown out of proportion in an epic way. He was angry that it was crippling his lifestyle and freedom to come and go as he pleased.

Mike claimed he was young, and that the youth didn't suffer from this thing. He was insistent that he didn't need to do video sessions that he should be allowed to come into my office. I reminded him that he could be a carrier and harm me, or I could be a carrier and he'd bring the virus to his elderly family relatives.

Roslyn, who feared the world was coming to an end, was in her seventies. Mike, on the other hand, felt he would live forever, and that this disease was for the old not the young. Mike was twenty. The fear of death impacts people in different ways at different times of their lives, depending on what's going on currently for them or due to their past experiences. Different ages — different perspectives — make humans look at scenarios through different lenses.

Day after day, month after month, I worked at the office, completely alone, as the other practitioners chose to work remotely from home, due to the coronavirus. I chose to have video sessions from my office to give the comfort of familiar surroundings to my patients. I wanted to create some type of norm.

Alone at the office, I found the atmosphere a bit quiet. I missed the hustle-bustle from the front desk, the phones' nonstop ringing and the reception room brimming with patients waiting, the soft music playing throughout. The place was silent.

Yearning for People

So after work, hungry for people, even if only from afar, I went for long, leisurely bike rides, as summer

97

nights remained light later with the time change. I was taking advantage of the opportunity to enjoy some fresh air. Most people those days were staying confined—or working, like I was, alone in an office without outside connection.

During one of my leisurely rides I cycled past a house lit with action—a party was going on. I could see heads bobbing up and down over the fence as they swayed to the music. I thought this was odd as we were counseled to not join in large gatherings—to congregate with no more than ten people at one time.

The next day I rode my bike the same way, and again to my surprise, a big bash of a party was in motion...at the same house. I heard music and laughter, and the driveway was populated with enough cars to make the place look like a used car lot. I was perplexed as everyone knew a distance of six feet was advised, and the get-together didn't sound limited to ten people only. Upon a closer look, I realized those together here were young adults partying heartily. *It's a party,* I mused to myself, but this wasn't the time to assemble, given the warnings.

So what gives, why would wall-to-wall people come together in a day-after-day gathering when we were told by the medical experts not to congregate? Spring break, I realized!! South Florida where the sandy beaches, bars, and restaurants are plentiful had become a mecca for students making the pilgrimage for a week of fun in the sun—and memorable and wild mistakes.

Young and fun all melded together for the spring breakers, and for a moment I missed that. To be young and carefree no matter what was going on, even a pandemic of this magnitude, certainly had its appeal.

Pedaling by, hearing Justin Timberlake swooning "Can't Stop the Feeling"...laughter and clinking of glasses, feeling the vibe of freedom as only carefree youth can enjoy, I knew what pleasure they were having. Song after song, beat after beat, mixed with the singing of the birds, fresh air, and the smell of the salty ocean breeze.

Perhaps the fear of death and dying is not as pronounced in the young because they can't wrap their heads around it, having, they believe, so much life ahead of them. Perhaps they aren't chasing youth because they are youth itself. For a split second or two, I was envious of the carefree youngness, as free as the wind.

Boom, boom, boom, the beat of Beyoncé, Taylor Swift, and Major Lazer's Jamaican-American electronic dance music, and Justin Bieber, to name a few I recognized, and others I didn't recognize, seared the air with one tune after the other.

For a moment I was caught up with the thought of endless partying, untroubled moments, drinking and flirting, and who knew what else. Ah, to be in the springtime of life. At that moment, I deliberated how they could throw caution to the wind when a pandemic was sweeping the world. I came to the conclusion that unless they'd come close to death from personal experience or the loss of a loved one, they would think they're untouchable.

So then the next day, forgetting about all the young and fun in the sun, I took a nice long morning walk with Southern Grace, my white Swiss shepherd, listening to Joanna Penn's podcast, *The Creative Penn Podcast*. This episode on writing was "How to Focus And Be Indistractable with Nir Eyal," featured on January 13, 2020.

Soaking it all in, the topic how *not* to get distracted, when I did just that—my attention diverted as a black Honda Civic screeched to a halt. A woman driving, wearing a black facemask, with two passengers in the back seat, slowed to a stop. At this point I hadn't seen anyone in Florida wearing masks with the exception of medical personnel. I was startled and scared, imagining all sorts of scenarios.

This eerie scene unfolded as I witnessed two young people exit the car, and the guy and girl who appeared to be in their twenties walk to that *very* house which was STILL populated with tons of cars and goings on in the yard, balcony, and inside the home. Every inch of the household was crowded with people. Again, I could see the top of their heads bobbing up and down as I peered through the occasional half-inch gap of each fence panel. I was again perplexed.

That evening, the reports on the news indicated many college parties were going on for spring break, suggesting the millennials weren't heeding warnings or recommendations to stay home and isolate. All curfews seemed to be ignored. I put two and two together, surmising this was a college spring break gathering—either with the parents away or it was a rental or airbnb.

Later, I learned the sprawling estate was leased as a "party house," rented weekly and on weekends for large gatherings. For sure, I wasn't sensing a fear of dying from this crowd. A continuous flow of people was coming and going.

Alone—the New Norm

While I'm writing this piece, I'm in my office on an early Thursday evening, and the space is quiet. No sounds. Usually a psychiatrist, a therapist or two, and others occupying offices are here, the waiting room bubbling over with people. Not today. I'm alone. All the professionals are working from home.

I chose to work in the office since I wouldn't have any more traffic than one patient at a time, if that. Initially, I chose to mix patients coming to the office and those I was seeing on video sessions. For the few who wanted in-person sessions, I finished five minutes ahead of schedule to avoid having patients in the waiting room. They waited instead in the car, and I texted when I was ready. I rushed to Lysol the leather couch and doorknobs.

This plan was squashed when patients became terrified to leave home, and I, too, became concerned about having a few straggling in who might not be following the distance recommendations.

Nearly every patient, however, preferred a video session, because they were at a heightened sense of fear they'd "catch" something and die a horrible death. Some patients were so terrified they wouldn't leave their homes, not for any reason, while others had compromised immune systems, and their doctors advised them to stay home. Such decisions were okay, too. The field of mental health care was considered "essential," and our associations advised working out the different options.

Some patients opted not to continue the therapy at all. But this group of non-attendees on any format was fewer than a few by finger count. Most of my caseload preferred to talk to me over video, phone, and lastly only a couple in person because the fear was great and real. Death and dying became a constant thought for many. And if it wasn't their death they worried about, they fretted over the death or possible death of someone they loved.

So as I sat alone in the eerily quiet office setting, listening to the birds chirping, with no sounds of cars or life out there, I considered death and dying, and aging, and the expectations, as we grow older. I never factored in a pandemic such as this when I began this book. I never thought of the entire world on lockdown of some sort, waiting to move on with life.

As the days passed, the pandemic grew and grew, and so did the fear. Though activity in some sense slowed down, my neighbors became more and more involved with activities outside, like biking, walking, and skating—all with the "six feet" of designated space, and with us only nodding a hello to our neighbors and moving on.

At this point, most donned the mask. When I happened upon *the house* once again, it was totally empty with enough garbage ready for pickup to fill an entire condo from floor to ceiling. I scanned the contents from my vantage point only to view empty Heineken bottles, Budweiser, bottles of whiskey, vodka, gin, sodas, and plastic cups. A hoedown for sure had taken place here for days on end, party attendees negligent of the fact we were at the onset of a full-blown pandemic. Yet I almost longed to hear the music and see the heads bopping up and down again—as if all was okay—even though it wasn't.

So after all that we've been through with this virus—my prayer is by the time you read this it has come and gone—I do wonder what your thoughts were about death and dying during such a time. And where are you now in regard to living your life? Einstein says we have only two ways to live our lives. One is as though nothing is a miracle. And the other is as though everything is. Which way do you live? Which way do you choose?

During the onset of such a frightening world crisis, did you think about your own death? As I noted earlier, I had one patient, Roselyn, certain the entire world was coming to an end, while the young fellow, Mike, was quite nonchalant about the whole thing. Was it that he was young, and this virus was killing mostly the elder? Maybe. But in time the younger man, too, will contemplate dying as it's happening around us and is soon to touch him in some way. Perhaps he's better off in his jolly state of mind, as most of my young patients are, as youth seems to be a forever thing...but it's not.

When Death Comes Knocking

For all of us death and dying are inevitable. We can entertain the idea with fear or with open arms. I prefer to accept with open arms. Perhaps we can consider steps to take to look at death and dying with an open mind.

I've been reading a book by Ann Richardson, *Life in a Hospice: Reflections on Caring for the Dying*, which opened my eyes from the caretaker's view as well as that of the recipients of such care. In the foreword, Tony Benn, a passionate supporter of the hospice movement, writes, "My mother, a very religious woman, said death is God's last and greatest gift to the living."

But how could God's greatest gift be death? Possibly the remark stems from a belief that life goes on, that life is more than our existence on earth, that we are not of this world. Or the idea of death being a gift could be coming from the fact that death can offer the relief of long-term pain or perhaps provides a transition from loneliness because loved ones and friends are no longer here.

Mr. Benn goes on to say, "The more I think about the hospice movement, the more I feel the issue is not *dying* well, but *living* well until you die." This says it all. I think over the idea of living well as assisting in dying well. Food nutrition and spiritual nutrition sprinkled with a healthy lifestyle of moderate exercise, loads of drinking water, play, and laughter all contribute to living well — so that we can die well. Yes, that makes sense.

Susannah Cahalan wrote a gripping memoir about a medical mystery, *Brain on Fire*, a powerful account of one woman's struggle to recapture her young, full life as it was. She was working at the *New York Post* when her career was momentarily interrupted by an illness that almost left her for dead. The book is a fascinating look at a disease that could have cost this vibrant, vital young woman her life.

Some initial diagnosis focused on the possibility that maybe Susannah had cancer since she'd had a brush with it earlier, having melanoma. After a series of tests, exams, probing, and multiple seizures, her doctors learned Susannah had anti-NMDA-receptor encephalitis, a multistage disease that varies widely in its presentation as it progresses.

In Susannah's case, her speech, thoughts, and movements, not to mention what were thought to be psychiatric issues, appeared as symptoms until the neurologists were called in to uncover the real problem. Youth as she knew it, changed for her, but for most of us youth is youth, and death and dying are far, far away.

Brain on Fire reminded me of Marilyn, a friend I worked with when I tended bar and she served drinks. She had a rare blood cancer that eventually claimed her life in her twenties, but she made her life work until her very last breath. She was courageous and strong and beyond her years in wisdom. She lived her life as though everything was a miracle.

Journalist Susannah Cahalan and my friend Marilyn were close in age, both in their twenties, both fearing death, and both dealt with cancer and other diseases — one died and one lived — a lesson for all that youth can be snatched at a moment's notice.

"There are only two ways to live your life. One is as though nothing is a miracle. The other, as if everything is." ~Albert Einstein. Miracles come in all sizes, shapes, and colors. Live your life as if everything is a miracle, and watch the magic happen.

So as we age, death and dying are in the background for most and foreground for some, but for those chasing youth, they do so as a way of pushing away the inevitable — at least for the moment. Is postponing death possible — pushing it far back? Perhaps our genetic codes can answer this question. Or maybe our lifestyles can advance or put off our time of death. Chapter Seven examines the age-old question of genetics versus lifestyle.

Personal Inventory Questions

1. "There are only two ways to live your life. One is as though nothing is a miracle. The other as if everything is." ~Albert Einstein. How do you live your life?

2. Most people don't think about death or the fear of dying with intensity until it is peering around the corner, either from the loss of a loved one, or due

to an illness we are battling. When did you become aware of death and dying — or have you not yet? And how does aging factor in?

3. This mysterious virus came to us by many names but seemed to settle with the novel coronavirus being known as COVID-19. COVID-19 soon became the subject of non-stop chatter as it moved in on all parts of the world. Did the virus pull you away from your aging concerns, or catapult you into deeper obsessions about aging?

4. One anxious patient, Roslyn, feared this was the end of the world — we were all going to die. She was scared. Prior to the virus pandemic, Roslyn was focused on aging and cosmetic surgery. Did the pandemic steer you, too, away from your previous concerns? Did those issues return as the pandemic where you live simmered down? What did you learn about yourself during this time?

5. Not every patient took the situation in the same spirit; some were nonchalant like Mike, a strong construction-worker fellow who refused to believe this virus was *that* serious. Mike was in his twenties with his whole life in front of him and that's all he could see. Do you think youth prevents us from seeing?

6. Ann Richardson's, *Life In A Hospice: Reflections on Caring for the Dying,* is a book from the caretaker's view as well as that of the recipients of care. The foreword, written by Tony Benn, a passionate supporter of the hospice movement, notes, "My mother, a very religious woman, said death is

God's last and greatest gift to the living." What do you think about that? Is that the great final miracle for us on Earth?

7. Many of us worked remotely during the pandemic, missing outside connections. This is perhaps what happened for you, too. How did you work through your alone time? Did you self-reflect about plans going forward?

8. South Florida where the sandy beaches, bars, and restaurants are plentiful has become a mecca for students making a pilgrimage for a week of fun in the sun — a time of memorable and wild mistakes as spring break ensues. Did you take spring break in your college days? Young and fun meld together for the spring breakers. Do you miss that?

9. Susannah Cahalan and my friend Marilyn were close in age, both in their twenties, both fearing death, both having dealt with cancer and other diseases — one died and one lived — a lesson for all that youth can be snatched at a moment's notice. Did you lose your youth early in life? Did it change your perspective on aging?

10. What lessons have you learned about death and dying at this stage of your life? Does aging factor in? What about the obsession with aging?

Chapter 7

Genetics vs. Lifestyle

Do not wish to be anything but what you are,
And try to be that perfectly.
~St. Francis of De Sales

Wishing to be only what you are and trying to be *that* perfectly—especially when chasing the impossible challenges of youth and perfection—is not so easy. The worldwide expectation of us seems to be that we ought to wish to be anything but what we are. If our hair is straight, the fashion of the day wants it curly; blond…well we're called upon to make it brunette; dark skin? heck let's make it lighter—and on and on, we chase being anything but what we truly are.

Yet the fact of the matter is being our best is being who we were born to be. If a divine source governs the universe, then all was written in the stars long before we arrived on Planet Earth. How we will age is perhaps up to the individual, but some parts of us, internally and externally, were set all along through our deoxyribonucleic acid (DNA), which is a self-replicating material present in nearly all living organisms as the main constituent of chromosomes. In fact, DNA is the carrier of genetic information, which was put in place long, long ago.

We will age, as a given, but how we age is a different story. Some of us age gracefully while others do not. The question is why? Why do some people age "well"? I'm sure you've known at least one person who maintained their youthful appearance and mannerisms well into the aging process, while others seemed old looking and acting, when in fact, they were still quite young. This divergence in the aging process is a mystery perhaps, or maybe not. You decide from your point of view as you plug in the information below while we examine the effect of genetics versus lifestyle.

For sure, nobody likes having wrinkly skin or doing the "old persons" shuffle, but eventually everyone will undergo the process of aging. Inevitably, as we grow older, our bodies and minds, inside and out, begin to change. Though seeing the physical changes in our bodies from the inside is harder than seeing aging in the mirror, the result of the passage of time IS happening internally *and* externally, simultaneously.

Genetics or Environment?

Though this change caused by the passage of the years is coming, some people tend to age more slowly than others. Why is that? Well, the cause is two-fold, both genetic and environmental; the influence of each causes the changes. Some of the factors that impact aging, such as lifestyle, are within our control, while genetics may not be.

If our parents were short, we have a good chance of being short, too, unless we also have an uncle or great uncle, aunt, grandpa, or so on, who was tall. Or we might have red hair or red hues as does Great Aunt Betty who was a carrot top, showing the family genetic code had such a potential in its distribution.

I actually have an Aunt Betty, long passed, who was a red-headed spitfire, a high-spirited, gutsy woman, fearless enough to leave her well-known, influential high-society newspaper family behind in Wisconsin. Instead, she made her way to Florida to marry a dashing airline pilot.

Back then for a woman to leave her home and move far away and marry a pilot was a very, very big deal. And for someone to be a pilot, in and of itself, was unique. Airplanes as a mode of travel weren't commonplace the way they are now. Flying in a plane was something many were in awe of — or afraid of — at the time.

As for genetics, Aunt Betty inherited the red hair from my Great, Great Aunt Mary, who was a redhead, and also a spitfire, who lied about her age so she could join the military, and then was stationed in

111

Alaska. Again, a big step for a woman back in those times to up and leave home and travel alone to unfamiliar parts.

One time many, many years ago, I was on a weekend visit to see my mom in Wisconsin. While upstairs in her country home, I noticed she displayed a wide array of pictures on the wall, pictures of her parents and some other family members, including one of me and my small son. How in the world did I make the cut when the pictures were generations and more above me, I wondered. I actually couldn't recall when the one of Benjamin and me had been taken. I was sitting outside in a lounge chair, and he was two-ish on the chair with me.

I stared intently at that picture, considering when it had been taken—and where had I been? And wow, I didn't remember ever wearing a crisp white shirt with black buttons and black cotton pants with an elegant white pair of tennis shoes—and little Benjamin all in white. I didn't recall looking so gracefully refined and dignified in Wautoma, outside surrounded by red and white pine and white spruce trees.

The photo seemed so not like me. Benjamin and I were sitting so appropriately in a wide wooden chair, the little tyke on my lap, looking up at the blue sky.

Mom broke the spell when she happened to come stand behind me. "Oh, do you like the pictures I put up?" she asked.

"Yes, they're amazing. When did you take the one of me and Benjamin? I don't recall."

112

Wautoma winters are brutally cold, so for sure the setting was summer, near the main house. I couldn't quite remember the pungent scent of pine and sap, sounds of lightening bugs buzzing by, and summer perennials with orange lilies scattered about, plus probably smacking at mosquitoes and hearing crickets and insect sounds of summer unfolding.

I would have remembered slapping at the mosquitoes, as they loved to bite into my flesh. I would have remembered us hidden deep within the tall trees—breathing in the sap-filled air of hundred-year-old pines. I would have remembered their needles spread over the earth, often pricking my bare feet when I ran down to the lake across the rock slabs (used as makeshift steps), often stubbing my toes.

No, this didn't seem a day I could pull together in my mind, try as I might.

And to my surprise, Mom responded, "That's not you, Lisa, that's your Aunt Betty, and the boy is your cousin Mike!"

I was astounded. The photo looked *exactly* like me and *exactly* like Benjamin. How could that be? How could I for certain identify myself, and the little guy in a picture and it not be us? The reason is genetics. In that photo, my Aunt Betty looked just like me, and baby Mike bore a close resemblance to Benjamin.

What are genetics? On a basic level, the science of genetics is the study of heredity in general and of genes in particular. The science of genetics looks into the gene pool, which plays a huge role in our internal and external happenings.

Molecular genetics focuses on the role of DNA, RNA, proteins, and other molecules in expressing the information stored in the genetic code. A gene is a particular stretch of DNA that codes for a certain trait. The genome is the complete complement of genes stored in an organism's cells.

Though our genetic code may be a given, we can control the environment we live in once we enter the adult world. We can manipulate our aging process and how we look, but genetics seem tough to undo. Following the lifestyle path, on the other hand, we can avoid such aging effects that come from direct exposure to the sun, excessive alcohol, poor quality foods, lack of sleep, drug abuse, and anger—yes even anger causes stress, which induces aging.

But as to the matter of genetics, is it true that we can't escape heart disease, cancer, diabetes, and such that run in the family? My mother's father, uncle, and father-in-law all passed away without warning from heart attacks. Was the cause genetics, or lifestyle? Or even something else—belief? The answer is really not clear-cut. Perhaps the genes may have been triggered, or perhaps as Bruce Lipton PhD, a developmental biologist, suggests in his book *The Biology of Belief,* even the idea that our genes will produce a certain fatal disease can be what causes that illness to bloom.

Though some flaw of ours seems genetic, perhaps the idea of the flaw was powerful enough to create it in the body—or perhaps some harmful lifestyle was passed down.

And, of course, as we age, our immune system function does decline. Doctors call it immunosenescene, a natural tendency toward diminished immunity as we age. We know this by comparing pictures of ourselves, and others taken ten years apart. We'll see our aging process in our face, skin, and hair color. This diminished immunity is the effect of age or the accumulation of toxins due to lifestyle, or a belief in the effects of aging, or a combination of all three.

What's mysterious may be the difference in rate of decline between individuals, though inevitably we all decline at some point. Our bodies simply don't produce as many immune cells as we grow older.

I knew a family where the grandparents and their kids and their kids' kids all had cancers of some sort. Either something was in the water or the air, or the cause was genetic. My first guess would be a genetic basis to the disease. But also, of course, smoking and drinking and poor quality foods can be common causes within a family, which means the triggers may have been environmental. Moreover, a belief in the inevitability of a certain disease catching up with us may invite its advent.

Science notes, too, certain locales have out-of-the-norm cases of cancer — presumably environmental due to toxic dumps. Often the source of particular diseases comes from a combination of factors, but sometimes not.

This aging is a slow process that takes time; just as our immune system function slowly declines.

What's mysterious may be the difference in rate of decline between individuals, but inevitably we all decline at some point. Our bodies simply don't produce as many immune cells as we get older.

Aiden's Journey

One day, Aiden, a charismatic fellow, called me out of the blue, wanting my hypnosis services. He wanted me to hypnotize him not to drink. He was insistent that he's not an alcoholic but enjoyed drinking and found slowing down difficult once he started. I gently explained if an alcoholic gene is lurking or a chemical imbalance of some sort lies beneath the alcohol problem, mere hypnosis wouldn't work. Aiden insisted that wasn't his situation, but that he simply wanted to slow down his drinking.

I was taken aback when I first met my new patient because his age didn't match his face; he looked many years beyond his actual years. Against my better judgment, we proceeded with the hypnosis. He was determined to be a casual, social drinker and not a spree drinker. Life without a cocktail or a glass of wine with dinner or a beer after a long day at the beach seemed incomprehensible to him.

And so we went along with hypnotherapy. And after several rounds of hypnosis, Aiden accepted that he wasn't snuffing out the addiction. The drinking only seemed to increase, with many poor choices and blackouts.

So, my patient and I regrouped and worked on cognitive behavioral therapy to massage and redirect the thinking and the behavior. We addressed the addiction component while the patient tapped into Alcoholics Anonymous after in-house treatment and rehabilitation, followed by intense out-patient work. Aiden began to understand alcoholism, and that he was an alcoholic who must stop drinking if he wanted to live a long and healthy life.

My patient's recovery was a process—a very long, three steps forward and two backward kind of road. And after the drinking since teenage years, along with dabbling in cocaine, not to mention loads of sun and fun sailing on the ocean, his skin had suffered for the worse too, his aging process catapulted a good fifteen years beyond his actual age. Aiden also prided himself on the fact that he operated on four hours of sleep, pushing his body beyond its natural limits.

One session, Aiden arrived full of despair, feeling he'd made little progress as the alcohol call gripped him. He was frightened, realizing this was bigger than him. At his AA meeting, he was reminded often that he needed to turn the problem over to God—his higher power. Yet he resented religion because his parents were obsessed with religion to the point he felt they were so busy churchgoing, they ignored actual spiritual growth. He struggled with God while not grasping any deep, permanent security or sense of intrinsic worth.

At some point, we took up the discussion of genetics versus environment. While Aiden was attending one of his Alcoholics Anonymous meetings, an acquaintance told him that he couldn't put the blame on genetics, that he was just making excuses. This was disturbing to Aiden because, in actuality, his family background wasn't one of drinking; in fact, his parents and relatives never drank, not ever. They were churchgoers and non-partiers. He had become defiant at a very young age—twelve, to be exact, which was when he started to drink.

So I began to scratch my head, wondering what was going on with Aiden. Well, one teeny tiny fact that Aiden failed to mention early on in his therapy was that he was adopted. As with many who are adopted, he felt shame, a shame at not being wanted, thrown out, so to speak, so he never disclosed this small detail.

But once his dark secret was out, Aiden began to search for his birth parents, only to learn they both were deceased, having died from complications of excessive drinking. Voila! He now was able to track the alcohol gene and to learn other things about how he was aging.

I wondered why Aiden was so secretive about his adoption, if maybe the family had a taboo against discussing it. I learned he overheard his dad tell a family acquaintance that *all* of his children were adopted—all five. And from different families, because they wanted to help children left behind. Instead of having children of their own, they began a mission to rescue and adopt as many children as they could. They were fostering and adopting all of God's children.

Aiden was stunned and hurt that nobody had told him he was adopted. Up to that point, he thought his family seemed so perfect. So when he learned of his adoption he was knocked off balance. His whole life felt like a lie. He was twelve, the age at which he began to change.

After much exploration of both his birth family and the family who brought him up, Aiden began to put the pieces together, building his self-esteem. The happy ending is that Aiden no longer drinks; he's a health advocate and life coach, and looks fabulous today. He actually looks ten years younger than his age now. He sleeps seven hours instead of four; changed his foods from drive-thru fast food to natural, whole foods; tapped into his spiritual self; engaged in a local Events and Adventure social club; and bloomed into the spectacular oak tree he was meant to be all along.

Aging Is a Privilege

To age is not forbidden, because with advanced age comes maturity, wisdom, and a wealth of experience that money and youth can't acquire. Ah, but to be thirty, with the wisdom of a seventy-year-old would be quite the elixir. But for most of us to have the wisdom that only life's journey of ups and downs grants, and yet to be young isn't possible.

Aging is like a fine wine — the more we age, the better we can become as a person. But we want to look good too. We want to be that wise person who is fit in body and mind.

No doubt environment and genetics play a huge role in the process of aging as we saw with Aiden, but so does money. Money doesn't buy happiness, but it can give a step up for those who purchase products to slow down the aging or make us look younger. Money can downshift the aging process in that it may grant more opportunity for finer foods, better doctors and insurance, as well as education, all of which *could* make a difference in the speed of the aging process. Money can also afford the person surgeries, fancy creams, salves, and potions.

Though we are set with our genetics, we can take some measures to turn back the clock. We have no guarantee that no matter what we do we'll live a long life, but perhaps some treatments might make a difference in how we age. Some are fortunate to rely on their bodies to tap into their human growth hormone to change the pace of aging. Others may need help.

Growth hormones, peptide hormones that stimulate growth, cell reproduction, and cell regeneration, is a topic we'll explore a bit through a non-medical lens. Growth hormone or somatotropin, also known as human growth hormone, stimulates growth in humans and animals. Human Growth Hormone (HGH) is produced by the pituitary gland.

Human growth hormone is a natural hormone produced by the body. It is a polypeptide, or a chain of amino acids that ignite growth of the cells. HGH also helps in cell repair and regeneration. Most notably, in order to enhance the growth of our muscles and bones, we need HGH.

Though HGH can be a good option, as with any procedure, we always risk a possibility of some side effects, such as nerve, muscle, or joint pain, along with swelling due to fluid in the body's tissues (edema), carpal tunnel syndrome, numbness, and tingling of the skin.

I recall a young patient, Bobby, who wasn't growing at the rate of his classmates. Bobby first came for sessions because he was self-conscious and insecure. He was distraught and obsessed with his weight and his short stature. He begged his parents to do something, but they feared the consequences of medication for their young pre-teen.

Yet in time, with some prompting, they finally agreed to look into options for their son. Bobby's father, a general practitioner, had many doctor friends with whom he could discuss the possibilities going forward.

The need for growth hormone for children is almost always diagnosed and prescribed by an endocrinologist. Endocrinology is the medical practice that specializes in diseases or defects of the endocrine system. After research and interviewing many doctors, Bobby's parents took him to such a specialist, and he began HGH treatments.

In order to enhance the growth of our muscles and bones, we need human growth hormone. HGH helps the body to gain muscle and develop denser bones in order for us to be taller and stronger. In addition, the hormone plays a major role in protein synthesis. Furthermore, HGH stimulates the breaking down of fats stored in the body. In time, Bobby began to grow and thin out.

This hot little ticket, human growth hormone, is not only for the teen who's not growing, but can also attract attention from the older population who want to slow down the aging process. It is quite popular today in creams, gels, pills, etc.

Why is HGH so sought after by adults? Well, the answer is simple, it works to slow down and repair the natural decline with aging. And the hormone is something our bodies naturally use anyway. I found myself pulled into the wonders of what human growth hormone could actually do for someone aging…though in a natural way.

But before we tap into human growth hormone through products, I want to mention that most people don't know that a wide variety of foods can naturally increase human growth hormone. Studies show foods can stimulate the production of growth hormones in the body. Glutamine is an amino acid that plays a huge role in the production of protein and building muscles as well as serving as a good source of energy. It can be found in pork, beef, fish, cheese, and milk products. It can also be found in raw vegetables, as well as beans.

In addition to glutamine, foods such as pineapples and coconut oil can trigger production of the hormone, along with goji berries. And of course, lots of water along with sleep and exercise can support growth spurts and body development. As discussed above, human growth hormone is produced by the pituitary gland and plays a key role in growth, body composition, cell repair, and metabolism.

This amazing growth hormone also boosts muscle growth, strength, and exercise performance, while helping us recover from injury and disease. Sounds like a miracle potion, doesn't it? It can be—and our diet and lifestyle choices can significantly affect our human growth hormone levels.

As I began to turn the corner in my own aging process, I started to look for a way to feel healthier and more youthful overall as my joints were becoming creaky and achy, especially my left knee. Also, I type up patient notes and write books, and my hands had begun to cramp. Most important, I watched an acquaintance morph into a happier, more youthful person after she began using a human growth hormone transdermal gel for a good eight months. She changed.

She became less agitated, less defensive, and more peaceful. Her face began to glow and her eyes had a sparkle I hadn't seen before. She seemed happier and steadier emotionally. She no longer practiced destructive behavior such as drinking, smoking, and misusing prescription drugs.

No, this wasn't an overnight miracle by any means. She started psychotherapy working with a psychiatrist, attended self-help and motivational groups, and in time, a new person came to light. She wanted and subsequently manifested a better self. She had alcoholism and depression to contend with, along with poor environmental choices that rocked her world — and not for the better.

But my friend made environmental changes in her life, such as eating healthy by choosing natural, unprocessed foods; she practiced yoga and took long walks; and she meditated and turned to a spiritual practice. She turned away from cocktails and began to drink water, something she had despised but learned to love. She transformed from a bitter, guarded, irrational, and fearful person into a warm, loving, rational, trusting human being.

Her change piqued my interest. I liked what I saw and inquired what she was doing. Most of her changes, I had implemented years and years before when I began my recovery from food addiction and binge eating disorder, but I wanted to look and feel fresher and become more mobile and less achy. I wanted something safe and natural that my body would produce on its own, with a little prompting. And I thought perhaps I had found it. I was surprised at the noticeable changes in my friend and wanted the same transformation, too.

I have chronic fatigue syndrome (an autoimmune deficiency) and arthritis, and soon saw a measurable change in both. Further, due to my having periodontal disease, I'd had one of four quadrants of gum surgery prior to using the gel — with the other three quadrants scheduled. But using the gel, I was able to forgo the additional three surgeries because I no longer needed gum grafts. I found that with this natural gel, along with not eating sugar, flour, or wheat; exercising moderately daily; drinking plenty of water; and enjoying a decent amount of sleep, I felt more youthful, and my skin took on a healthier glow.

I'm not going to promote this gel as that's not the importance of this book, it's just a sidebar, and those of you who know me know I'm transparent and authentic, and if I'm doing something that enhances my quality of life, I'll share it with you. And with that, I say, take what you need, and leave the rest. We all are searching for our optimal life, and using whatever natural means to get there should be the quest.

So, we can consider changing the environment we live in and making a difference, or changing a potential threat of genetics through changing our lifestyle. Look at Aiden; he's now a prosperous life coach abstaining from alcohol and looking years younger than his natural age. And then I think of little Bobby, not so little anymore, whose genetics produced short family stature, and now he's a tall, handsome, productive artist living in California. And then my friend, who transformed before my very eyes, impresses me.

We have choices to make in order to change and to live our best lives. Selecting our actions well is the start of the process. Don't wish to be anything but what you are, but try to be that perfectly — without obsession, so you can go on to live your authentic life, as we'll look at in Chapter 8.

Personal Inventory Questions

1. "Do not wish to be anything but what you are, and try to be that perfectly. There are only two ways to live your life." ~St. Francis of De Sales. Wishing to be only what you are and trying to be *that* perfectly — especially when chasing the impossible challenges of youth and perfection — is not so easy. What do you think?

2. We will age. Aging is a given, but how we age is a different story. Some age gracefully, while others do not. The question is why? Why is it some people age well, without stress? How do you think you're aging?

3. Though this change is coming, some people tend to age more slowly than others. Why is that? Well, the cause is two-fold, genetic and environmental; both influences cause the changes. Some of the factors that impact aging such as environmental are within our control, while genetics may not be. How has the environment played a role in your aging? What about genetics? Which is the greater influence?

4. When I learned the picture on the wall of my Great Aunt Betty was not of me, I was quite shocked, as the resemblance was uncanny — identical to the point I was certain the photo was of me. What features of yours do you find to be like those of one of your relatives? As you look at your family members, do you notice many

reminders of relatives you knew in the past in the features of relatives of today?

5.   We can do much to control our aging process and how we look, but genetics are tough to redo. We can avoid such things as direct exposure to the sun, excessive alcohol, poor quality foods, lack of sleep, drug abuse, and anger—yes even anger causes stress, which causes aging. But sometimes we can't escape heart disease, cancer, and diabetes that run in the family. What family medical history have you inherited? How is it impacting your aging process?

6.   Are you an Aiden? Do you carry a secret that's crippling your life? He hid his alcoholism from himself and pretended he wasn't adopted because both made him feel bad. But as you learned, we are only as sick as our secrets. He openly told on himself and now is blooming. What about you?

7.   Do you find natural foods boost your health? What foods make a difference with your skin and joints? Often we can pinpoint the culprits that keep us from living our healthiest best.

8.   I mentioned that money plays a role in defying age. What are your thoughts about that? Do you feel money is the only way to find youth? What ways have you changed naturally without spending money?

9.   I was looking for a way to feel healthier and more youthful overall as my bones were getting creaky and achy, especially my left knee. Also, I type notes on patients and write books, and my hands

began to cramp. I also watched someone morph into a happier more youthful person after she began using a transdermal gel for a good eight months. Who has influenced your positive changes?

10. Some people are fortunate to live a long life and even look young for their age, while others may begin to age early, before their time — and maybe not look youthful any longer. Do you have a family history of long lives and youthful presentation? What leads to that? How do you fit into that equation?

Part II

Realignment

Chapter 8

Living Your Authentic Life

How we spend our days is,
of course, how we spend our lives.
~Annie Dillard

If you were to attend your own funeral, what would you hear others saying about you? Would they describe you as a person living your authentic life? And what does living your authentic life look like for you? Living your authentic life as a person with maturity allows you to be you exactly as you are, but with more spit and fire, more courage, more wisdom than you could ever have had in your younger years. Why? Because this time you're armed with experience, something only age can provide. You're at an advantage now.

How you spend your days is, of course, how you spend your life. How are you spending your days? Do you close your eyes at night and give thanks, thinking, *It was good.* If not, this is an indication you aren't living your authentic life as YOU intended. And this is big, because this failure to live your authentic life leaves a gap for disappointment, opening the doors for depression, anger, and guilt. No worries though, because every day is a new opportunity for change, no matter your age, no matter the situation.

Living life on purpose is one of the greatest defenses against depression. Are you living your best life? I ask my patients this question during our initial session to take the temperature as to how they're spending their days, so I can grasp if they're living their lives on purpose. When I ask the question, I'm greeted with a stare. I know that stare because I had the same one many years ago. The stare says, *Are you kidding me? I can't live my authentic life because…*and you fill in the blank.

So the question is; how do you know if you're living your indisputable, true-to-yourself life? How do *you* know? You know by how you start your day and how you end your day. If you wake feeling you're facing a day of drudgery and resenting having to go to work, then you already have an inkling you're not on point. Not every day is a perfect day, but if every day starts off badly and ends badly, this is a sign you're not on the mark.

The other day I was scrambling to put together a blog due to a shortage of time, so I perused some of my very old blogs from long, long ago. I repurposed a blog of mine from nearly twenty years ago using a mission statement as to what I wanted to accomplish going forward. What follows is part of the blog.

Dream Big

One of my favorite pleasures in life was to sit in the "Florida Room" in my mom's home in Wautoma, Wisconsin. Early in the morning, I loved to go out to the octagon-shaped room surrounded by oblong windows, which gave an outdoor feel, with a mug of hot decaffeinated coffee, to sit in the silence. Deer and exotic birds always entertained me as I sat and looked out.

I liked to think of the Wisconsin Florida Room as a meditation space, an area where I became quiet with my thoughts, a place where I was in prayer — A place to be still, which gave me a sort of meditation/self-hypnosis feel.

Yes, I did say self-hypnosis. I find *self*-hypnosis to be one of the most powerful tools every person has access to. We can all sit quietly and go into the subconscious mind and implant suggestions that take hold.

The mind is powerful.

I can close my eyes, right here in South Florida as I type this piece, and go to the Florida Room in Wautoma and see those very same deer grazing and walking through the morning dew. I recall a glorious day that last time I was there, now so long ago! I felt completely serene and connected to the universe just looking out into the wide array of forest and open land. That was the very place I used to ride Pasha, my white Arabian, during my teenage years, looking for quiet and stillness.

On that last day (nearly twenty five years ago) in the Florida Room, I meditated and self-suggested my goals and aspirations, while ingesting the glory of the morning. I visualized where I wanted to be years from then. I imagined earning my doctorate in psychology, teaching at a university, and bringing my work to the internet, all while writing books in a way that could reach everyone.

I believed to the core of my being, but I had one "small" problem. I was in major debt from student loans and credit cards and I would need years and years to accomplish these dreams. Pushing away the negativity, I mapped the progression I so dearly longed for in that very room in a notebook, then closed my eyes and imagined my dreams were all possible if I put them out there in the universe. I prayed, and believed.

And Then I Let It Go — *Let Go, Let God...*
As you see, my wishes all came to fruition. And if it happened for me, it can happen for you, too. Of course the achievement of your goals isn't going to come to you as simply as by wishing on a star, but if you put your dreams in motion, they can emerge.

Think of the action you take like a reset, and watch the miracles unfold.

Back then, way back then, I knew I needed to craft a personal mission statement concerning what I wanted, and then let my hopes come to life.

As you might imagine, I work with patients who have many different needs, and one issue that often pops up is a disappointment that they aren't living their lives on purpose, coupled with the sense that "if only I were thinner, smarter, younger, luckier..." and on it goes....

They feel stuck.

To move forward and conquer fears, make a plan. Believe in something greater than you, and perhaps seek a therapist who can work with you through psychotherapy and self-hypnosis.

Psychotherapy begins where the patient presently is, with some poking into the past; and from there, we build dreams and opportunities. Sometimes I only use talk therapy with my patients, other times cognitive/behavioral therapy, and sometimes we explore self-hypnosis. Often we dive into a combination of all three.

Talk therapy is based on talking freely and gathering information for us to examine; cognitive behavioral therapy starts with looking at the thought process, the way a person thinks, while the behavioral aspect means changing or adjusting behavior to be more productive; and last, self-hypnosis starts with relaxing the patient and then making strong suggestions we both agree upon before hypnosis begins. All of these approaches work independently or in concert.

The treatment that receives the most attention is hypnosis. The idea that change can occur through suggestion alone is fascinating for most. Of course, a trained mind can relax and make dreams come to fruition on its own, the way I did way back in Wisconsin by meditating on my wishes, wants, and dreams.

I had a patient ask me the other day if I thought everyone could be hypnotized. After I considered the question for a moment, I answered yes, as long as the person isn't suffering from brain damage or severe mental illness. I think the big misunderstanding is that hypnosis means losing control over your mind, when in fact the result is actually the opposite. Rather, hypnosis helps you with the training of your mind so that you're able to enter a relaxed state and redirect your thinking.

Over my two decades of conducting hypnotherapy, I have seen remarkable results. The mind is an amazing faculty...and it will take you wherever you want to go with a little imagination and creativity. In fact, Chapter 17, ahead, is a fun chapter in which you can build your personal self-hypnosis/guided imagery script and imagine your ideal later years into reality.

Often when a patient comes to me for self-hypnosis, I ask them to find a place in their mind that brings them serenity, a place that is peaceful and safe. This setting you might visit could be as warm and fuzzy as a walk through a field of flowers, or a stroll barefoot on the beach feeling the warm sand between your toes—or curled up on a couch near the fireplace reading a good book with a crackling fire warming your feet—or for some, playing with puppies. *Everyone* has a place or two that brings such joy.

Another scene of serenity for me is remembering when I was a small child taking a nap on the back porch in Chicago with my dog, Cuddles. I can remember the smell of the closed-in porch and feel the breeze on my skin from the opened windows, bringing in the smell of cherry blossoms on a beautiful spring day. Those were magical, *easy* moments.

We all have a special place that allows us to embrace pure peace and harmony. And if you can't think of a real one, make it up! You can conjure one up from a picture in a magazine or a place you saw on television. The subconscious mind doesn't know the difference between real and pretend. For this reason, you can imagine yourself strong and vibrant, free of your aging obsession (or whatever concerns you have), and the mind will grab the image, even if it's not real...*yet*. Dream big!

I *knew* that magical morning in the Florida Room, my life was going to evolve to be even greater than it already was. I *knew* I was going to grow my practice beyond South Florida, teach at a university, and write books. And, in time, that's what happened—and is still happening. Just planting the seed and believing in my work set the wheels in motion.

Life for me is magical and promising. I feel as serene as the deer in the woods...living in the now...enjoying the moment. When my day is filled with busyness (and it often is), I close my eyes and go wherever I want my mind to take me. And of course one of my "getaways" is looking out at the wildlife from the Florida Room in Wautoma, Wisconsin.

Do you have dreams? If you could do anything you wanted what would it be? Do you find you're living the life you always dreamed of, or are you settling? Maybe you're doing fine, and that's amazing.

Whose Dream Are You Living?

Back in the day, in the Florida Room nearly thirty years ago, I was motivated by Steven Covey's inspiring book, *The 7 Habits of Highly Effective People: Powerful Lessons in Personal Change,* where he addresses developing self-awareness and how many of us "discover ineffective scripts, deeply embedded habits that are totally unworthy of us, totally incongruent with the things we really value in life."

This was certainly true of me, and of Chiara, whom you'll read about below—and most likely could be true of you as well. How do we find ourselves stuck in these ineffective scripts? The models may come from family, friends, teachers, rabbis, priests, and other influential people in our lives, but they might not spring from our own self-dreams and identities.

Perhaps you're living the life your mom or your dad wished upon you. Perhaps you didn't feel confident about doing what you *really* wanted to do. Our insecurities and self-doubts often get in the way and stop us from being our best selves. Do you do what you love and love what you do? Doing the work you love and loving what you do feels like play — the hours melt away without awareness because you're one with what you do.

Often I hear, "Why bother? I'm getting on in age — it's too late for me." No. It's never ever too late, unless you've taken a last breath — then it *is* done — at least here on the earth school. This is not to say no days are ever burdensome and no nights are filled with despair, because sometimes they are. But we can redirect. Stop a moment now, close your eyes, and take a realistic look at what you've done as of late, and I'm certain you'll find a list of accomplishments that have pleased you and about which you can say, "It was good."

Why build a list of good? Because building a list of good leads you to discover moments you can attribute to your very best self so you may better understand your own positive attributes. The list will assure you that you're genuinely a decent person with many great qualities. Start small. Who were you kind to as of late? Maybe you paid someone's car toll, or opened a door for someone, or went to the store for an elderly neighbor. What good deeds have you done? Find the smallest grain of good, and it will spark remembrances of more and more good things you've done.

And what made you happy? What fills your bliss tank?

When I was a small child, I used to dream about writing stories, but I never put that imagining into motion until later in life. I had the desire tucked away deep inside, but I left it there for that one, far-off day. And that's okay. Maybe I wasn't ready to begin my bliss, but I still was able to dip into other parts of my authentic self, and as I became stronger, I was able to take on more of my dreams to make them realities. We always can dip into the authentic "me," no matter what stage we're at and grow better able to take on the next step as we go.

We might start by building a mission statement. According to Covey, a personal mission statement based on correct principles becomes a personal constitution, the basis for making major, life-directing decisions. The personal mission statement can be the basis for making daily decisions in the midst of change.

I created exactly that sort of personal mission statement back in the Florida Room...when I knew I didn't want to be an attorney. I'd worked for a law firm as a paralegal, always feeling inadequate and out of place. I attended one semester of law school, and though I did well, the "fit" wasn't feeling right—but it sure pleased my father. His dream was to have a lawyer in the family.

And I really hoped to make my dad proud. I knew even then that I wanted to help people, yet not in a lawyer kind of way — but rather in a self-help, counseling way. I wanted to help build their confidence, self-esteem, and integrity, and find what made them giggle on the inside and outside at the same time.

I recall Chiara, a forty-something woman I worked with years ago, who had an unfortunate event occur in college that left her distraught. She'd partied hearty with a group of students who lived on the freshman floor of her dorm and passed out only to wake with several men taking advantage of her. Fear and disgust engulfed her — the disgust was for herself. She felt dirty and unworthy to live her best life.

Chiara quit school, and all her dreams went unfulfilled. By the time she reached me, she'd already dived into her eating disorder headfirst, filling all her moments focused on what to eat or not eat; exercise; and an obsession with arresting her aging. She blocked her authentic self as she jumped into marriage and family life, hoping it would erase the pain she'd tucked way back into her subconscious mind.

As time marched on, her girls grew, needing her less and less while her husband became more and more distanced. Chiara's two daughters, now teens, were on the verge of entering college, and needless to say, she was terrified they'd have an experience similar to hers. Once Chiara and I untangled her rational and irrational fears, we began to look at her life now and tap into what was missing. We also tapped into her tucked-away horror from long, long ago.

Chiara never told anyone, not anyone, about her college experience. She blamed her quick escape on anxiety and fled her college life where she'd begun to study social sciences and public administration. Chiara was a skilled communicator, often told she was a gifted storyteller, interning and volunteering in the fields of her passion. She dreamed of contributing to society and developing knowledge that could make a difference in the world.

Off Chiara went to Princeton University in New Jersey, a private Ivy League research university. Princeton, a far cry from her small town in Mississippi, offered a quiet town, familiar feel with the type of excellent education that would catapult her into the fulfillment of her aspirations. She walked the campus in disbelief that she'd finally made it to her dream school where she could immerse herself in research and make a difference. And then the vision ended in a nightmare before she had a chance to begin.

Fast forward. When I met her, Chiara wasn't living her authentic life because her eating disorder and obsession with aging stopped her from moving ahead. So we began our work with the eating disorder and what flamed it, unraveling the terrible college experience she'd never been treated for nor even told anyone about.

Chiara suffered from posttraumatic stress disorder, a mental health condition triggered by a horrendous event she'd experienced in college all those years before. She often had flashbacks, nightmares, and severe anxiety, as well as uncontrollable thoughts about that very night—or at least the parts she could remember.

Often in life, we're stuck with unresolved issues that throw us into another distraction to avoid the deep pain of facing an experience. If we go around rather than through the incident, long and lasting dysfunctional marks remain to plague us.

Chiara ate, dieted, restricted, and then ate again, compensating by over-exercising and indulging in a quest to stay young. And now, in this third act of her life, Chiara was questioning what her true calling was despite her being well into her fifties. Did she really want to try and pursue her research career? Just the thought of trying that made her feel anxious and uncomfortable.

Repeatedly, Chiara told me she felt too old. But I kept pushing and prodding because I wasn't sold on the idea that she wanted to be a researcher moving into a political realm. Chiara's father was an accomplished attorney, and her mom an administrator at a well-known school.

A given in the family was that Chiara would somehow follow in their footsteps with her communication skills and ability to research. Her parents had carved out what *they* thought would make her heart sing. But, it didn't. Yes, some unfortunate things happened at college years before, which truthfully can happen at any college, and does, but I saw that she also needed to deal with the fact she wasn't quite going after her authentic dream. Certainly, she wanted to change the world and give, but not quite in the way her parents had scripted for her.

We needed to dig deeper and look at what she'd blocked in her desires as a kid. What was her mission statement or list of wants? Come to find out that Chiara had spent years and years of her childhood molding dogs, cats, and birds out of clay. She loved the feel and the form as the blank slate of the material emerged into something from her imagination. But, no, that wasn't a *real* job; it was a hobby — according to her parents.

Chiara loved nature and God, and had a spiritual connection to the earth, sky, water, and all the blessings of life, including every creepy-crawler, bird, fish, and four-legged fur being. She was mesmerized by shows that discussed the planet and everything it entailed.

Finding all this out, I suggested perhaps she rekindle her love for sculpting and creating pieces that made people feel as connected to the earth as she herself felt. At first, she baulked at the idea, but soon the old passion of hers was lit. Today, Chiara, not too old to follow her inner instincts, makes pieces commissioned by many across the globe. She feels both authentic and alive.

How we spend our days is of course how we spend our lives. Are you living your authentic life? Tap into yourself and discover the treasures. Perhaps a mission statement or a list of your wishes and wants is a way to capture your true life script for you. And while you're at it, examine if you're an introvert or extrovert (Chapter 9) in your quest to become your authentic self.

Personal Inventory Questions

1. "How we spend our days is how we spend our lives." ~Annie Dillard. Are you spending your days according to the wishes of your deepest self?
2. If you were to attend your own funeral, what would you hear others say about you? Would they describe you as a person living your authentic life?
3. Living life on purpose is one of the greatest defenses against depression. Are you living your best life? I ask this question to my patients during our initial session to take the temperature on how they're spending their days, so I can grasp if they are living their life on purpose. Now I ask the question of you.
4. I work with patients who have many different needs and emotions, and one feeling that often pops up is a sense they aren't living their lives on purpose, coupled with "if only I were thinner, smarter, younger, luckier..." and on it goes. Are you stuck? Do you focus on physical appearances rather than your authentic self?

5. Do you have dreams? If you could do anything you wanted, what would it be? Do you find you're living the life you always hoped for, or are you settling?

6. Chiara suffered through an unfortunate event in college that left her distraught. Often we block or become trapped in the aftereffects of an incident that stays with us, shutting out our best life. Do you have a secret stopping you from living your life on purpose?

7. Have you ever created a mission statement for yourself as an individual subject? What would your mission statement look like if you created one today?

8. Back in my mom's Wisconsin Florida Room, I didn't look at all the obstacles in my way but rather let my mind run free with the idea I could be anything I wanted. I felt I could meditate and self-hypnotize my dreams into fruition. Do you believe you could? Have you? What's stopping you?

9. What was your favorite thing to do as a child? Did your parents support this activity? Do you today still engage in this favorite thing to do?

10. Do you feel too old to live your authentic life? What is the stop-age to becoming your best self? Who created this timeline? Is it true?

Chapter 9

Extrovert or Introvert?

If I am not for myself, who will be for me?
Yet if I am for myself alone,
of what good am I?
~Hillel the Elder

I woke with a start from a deep sleep in a slight panic with a knot burrowing in my stomach, a crippling worry that something was wrong—but what? My eyes popped open, and I stared out into the dark, wide-eyed, questioning what was disturbing my slumber. And then the COVID-19 came to mind—*our new norm.*

Life had changed, for the moment, as we'd known it, and hopefully by the time you read this book we've learned and grown much internally and externally from this pandemic experience. This is a time of isolation from others, a time to look within and reflect, and to look outward as to where we might want to take our lives going forward.

Some people have seemed relatively comfortable in the isolation, while others have struggled. For the introvert, this period has appeared to be an easier transition than for the extrovert, but I'm not certain. Perhaps the time has been challenging for both.

As we journey to our later years, we often become more particular regarding who we spend time with. Some friends have passed away, while others have moved. We may become more introverted or selective. And for most of us, the pandemic put a stop to interacting outside our homes or work, forcing isolation — time alone with self.

If I am not for myself, who will be for me? We do need to start with the internal self to be our best selves in order to help others. *Yet, if I am for myself alone, of what good am I?* For sure we count on strength in numbers — the whole world in this pandemic together, perhaps now forging through the unknown in unison, shifting us away from our inner, solo struggles, in order to reach out to others. But at the same time, the odd twist is that, yes, we're in this together, but simultaneously, we're distancing from each other. Odd indeed.

A Dance of Yin And Yang

We all have experienced a yearning for balance and normalcy as the weeks of isolation and social distancing ensued. This feeling could be labeled a yin and yang kind of movement. The often-seen yin-yang symbol, a circle made up of a black swirl and a white one, each containing a spot of the other, finds its roots in Taoism, an ancient Chinese philosophy.

The dark swirl represents the yin, which is associated with shadows, femininity, and the trough of a wave; the light swirl, represents the yang, meaning brightness, passion, and growth. The symbol as a whole stands for the light and the dark, day and night, good and evil, *young and old*—hence yin and yang.

The yin and yang, opposite forces, can be seen as interconnected and counterbalancing, which the introvert and extrovert dance between. People need people but also need time for introspection and self-reflection, which the lockdown forced on us. In isolation, we can't run or hide or block or numb out unless turning to the addictions—which many have used to escape this new norm.

But the healthier act is to reach out and touch others after first reaching in to find our balance—our own personal yin and yang. Of course, during this unparalleled time, reaching out and hugging and connecting physically has been forbidden, so talking through our smartphones and laptops, and by way of video chats has offered the virtual connection—without the hugs and warmth of a caring other.

I think of it as the clichéd oxygen mask rule on airplanes when the flight attendant instructs passengers to place the mask over themselves first so they can then help someone else. "Please place the mask over your own mouth and nose before assisting others" gives us a bizarre visual that makes us now think of donning cloth masks these days to protect ourselves, and each other, from the coronavirus. Strange to see, yet we're saving lives.

Is the introvert less able to assist others than the extrovert? Is the introvert less able to break free from the thoughts of aging than the extrovert? Or are both equally focused on their aging, regardless of whether they isolate or not? I'm meditating over this question as I'm now conducting sessions in a room, *alone,* with not another soul in the building—for going on to seven months.

I've noticed that the topic of aging and countering that with cosmetics and cosmetic procedures has been placed on the back burner for both the introverts and the extroverts. The focus has, instead, shifted to fears of becoming sick, being alone, and dying. But also the attention of many of my patients has moved to out-of-control eating, and many are making daily trips to the supermarket despite the advice to stay inside and prevent this virus from spreading.

I get it. Every day I've thought about making a quick run to the store, but common sense has prevailed, and I've refrained. I so understand the fear of running out of staples and being stuck. Wanting to *go out and buy*…whatever we might need…is human nature, even for an introvert.

One person, a self-proclaimed introvert, blurted out to me, "I'm out-of-control eating. I don't get it because I was doing *so* well. Now, my weight is inching up and I can't stand it. I'm afraid to leave my house, but I'm afraid to stay in. That's funny because normally, before this pandemic, I stayed in for days, and even weeks on end without any problem."

Six Feet Apart, yet So Close

So now we're disconnecting to connect through computers. Pre-coronavirus, I ranted on about how we're disconnecting to connect in an unnatural way, fearing we'll become less connected as human beings. But now, I'm taking a second glance and seeing how blessed we are to have the opportunity to connect— no matter from how far.

So, perhaps the internet has been part of the GREATER plan all along…

Maybe we were in training—a preparation so to speak—for now, as we socially disconnect in real-time, in the physical form, we've moved our real-time to connect through our computers and phones with emails, texting, etc.

Many are calling and texting, Facebooking and Face-timing with family they've not connected with in years. What makes people connect now? Where were they before? When in crisis, people apparently tend to reach out. Wanting to reach out when in the face of a fear life might come to an end is a very normal reaction. Every hurricane I've been through over the last 33 years proved no different. Always, without fail, family members from far away and friends I'd not heard from in a long time, call to connect.

Why?

Humans need humans. Though some of us are introverts, while others are extraverts, at some point we all need that human contact...knowing that someone out there is thinking about us, concerned if we're okay. Having to isolate at home is actually an opportunity to get out of the self and think of others.

The obsession over body changes begins to take a back seat as the fear of a real issue such as the coronavirus takes the front seat. But the reprieve is only for a short time, and all the while the nagging of aging is rumbling in the interior messaging of the mind.

A Song From Afar

As I was writing this section I sat under canopy on our swing, looking out at the water from time to time. Soon, a boat putt-putting and sputtering caught my attention as it maneuvered close to a dock across the way, with someone playing the most beautiful rendition of "Happy Birthday" I'd ever heard. Two people in the boat, elders, were serenading an even older man leaning on his cane looking out from his dock as the sun slipped behind the clouds, with his lovely wife by his side.

All the people from all the houses around went out on their docks and sang their neighbor a happy

90th birthday, *all aware of the distancing rule.* The event felt like something that would happen in Italy, with people singing from their patios, rooftops, and outside terraces while they were deep in the pandemic, with the virus taking so many lives...a lovely gesture indeed. *Another connecting of the disconnected...*

Disconnecting to Connect suggests we're social distancing more and more, even dating through the screen, but what if *that* was part of *this* greater plan — a God preparation. What if *this thing* was out there ready to strike and unbeknownst to us we were connecting long in advance through our devices as a preparation for things to come.

God Speaks

I'm hearing more talk about God these days than I've heard in a long time. Alone time is thinking time. Perhaps more self-reflecting has been in order with the worries of life coming to a close for some sooner than planned. I've had many tell me as of late during our video sessions that they're spending more quiet time than they'd ever done in their lives. One patient, Leonora, cried, pleading to come in for a session *just this one time* because she was so lonely — that the aloneness was unbearable.

This woman had never spent time alone like this with the exception of during her binge-eating days when she isolated during binge-eating manias. She was a very social person, otherwise, and work was her happy place — with lots of co-workers to share the gossip of the day with. Now she has been working remotely and said she was in her head all the time, thinking and worrying about what she was going to eat and when, and whether she had enough food, and how would she go to the store, when she was afraid that if she did, she might wind up catching the virus.

And the introverts have been saying something similar in that this is a *forced* alone time, which makes it different than the *preferred* alone time of *their* choice.

But now, even for the introvert, I've seen more connecting than ever before, a reconnecting and making amends through calls to long-lost friends during our 'shut-in" time. And Facebook is turning into a godsend for many — a platform inviting great suggestions.

One post that imprinted in my mind was passed around from LivingChristian.org: *While you wash your hands, PRAY for 20 seconds. Let's change the world!"* Can you imagine if everyone really did pray for 20 seconds, how many prayers would be sent out into the ether — the heavens? Think about how many times you've washed your hands today. Most of us have raw paws from the continuous washing.

One patient, Angel, who was quite social, who was always fearing her aging would take away her beauty, invested in a facelift, eyelift, and a tummy tuck, and feared any wrinkles of any type. But lately she has marveled at how that's not a concern for her right now, that her concern is her anxiety about what's going to happen next. The fear of the unknown has been what's crippling her. But of course she did mention when she goes out with her mask, she makes sure to highlight her eyes with mascara, eyeliner, and shadow, since that's the exposed part.

And then I think of Bessy, an introvert by nature, who ruminates about how she'll get by if her boyfriend of 13 years suddenly passes away from this virus. She no longer dwells on signs of growing old, but rather what to do if she's left alone without her life partner. This, of course, is another obsession with aging, though not from a vanity view but rather a left-alone view.

The fear for this patient of not being in control has been like fear on steroids in her mind, which conjures up one scary scenario after the other. I remind her that she and her significant other haven't left their home in weeks, that they're well stocked and in good health, so the chances of either one of them contracting this invisible enemy remains remote. I gently suggest she won't contract this virus if she stays put. And she does.

Quiet Can Be Deafening

Working in the quiet has been strange, really strange—no hustling bustling of patients in the waiting room, with doctors and therapists, receptionists, massage therapists, and other renters all no longer in the offices here. I'm alone—just me and my iPad screen placed in front of me on the desk looking into the eyes of the patient from their home, with my laptop on my lap capturing notes for their records. One after the other, a patient pops onto my screen. This is a new way of conducting sessions — with me, with the screen, with the laptop and the patient — alone — me on my end, and they on theirs.

I'm conducting ninety percent of my patient time through the computer via a video connect, and five percent by phone and five percent in person. So many of my introvert patients have let me in on a secret — that it's not so bad, this isolation, as they're used to it, that this is no different than their normal lives. Both the young and more mature patients begin to chat about their eating disorders, binge eating, and restricting, saying that these are worsening in their isolation — though the fact that some virus is pulsating and growing out there is not such a concern for the youth.

I marveled over that for quite some time. Many of my patients do separate from the rest of the world normally and aren't very social, but the difference is that now this type of situation is forced on them, and becomes uncomfortable, with the television blaring the message of doom and gloom for all. Before, their doom and gloom was fabricated in their minds, and their focus was on personal concerns. Yet for the younger ones the universal doom and gloom has almost seemed to enhance the emphasis on their personal concerns.

In addition to television coronavirus overdose, the time inside leads to more device time. During our later years, we may spend significant time on our devices, causing some distresses we're not aware of. Universal upsets may take over for all of us who isolate by choice or by force—the introvert and the extrovert—when diving into our devices. I list a few of the negatives of too much technology time below.

The Upsets of Remote Life

Sleep Disruption: Studies show use of electronics right before bed may stimulate you so that sleep becomes more elusive. At the same time, ninety percent of people in the US admit to using a device during the last hour before hitting the sack. Moreover, adults use electronic media to help them relax. But not only does the brain stimulation cause agitation, but also the light exposure is known to negatively impact sleep time, sleep quality, and even daytime alertness.

Poor Eating Habits: Grabbing snacky foods while engaged on our devices are easier than stopping all entertainment and sitting at a table to eat. Why? Well, we become bored only engaging in one activity. Today we multi-task rather than sit in the moment engaged with our food. Eating in a distracted way leads to overeating and/or choosing poor quality foods, because they're less time consuming to simply take from the kitchen and eat.

Stress: People who spend too much time online are at risk of depression and other mental illnesses. Spending long hours on your device of choice can disrupt the nervous system due to overstimulation, and causes the brain to be in a state of chronic stress.

Joint Aches: Sitting hunched over looking at a screen can lead to back pain and joint issues. Suffering from shoulder pain caused by the muscles and tendons between neck and wrist being held tensed in one posture for long periods is not uncommon. Again, we rarely sit upright when we're engaged on the computer or playing with our smartphones. We usually sit in a hunched-over position as we extend our necks out to see the screen. Poor posture at a device can also lead to wrist and finger joint pain...and carpal tunnel.

Sitting Too Much: Sitting too long can lead to varicose veins, or spider veins, and though these may not be harmful, they're not delightful to look at when you're wearing shorts or swimsuits. In rare cases, sitting too long can lead to more serious conditions like blood clots.

Withdrawal: Forced isolation can be lonely, especially for the extrovert, due to lack of social interaction. Social withdrawal and social isolation can make doing the things we normally would enjoy less likely.

Less Family Connection: When engaged online we may find ourselves reluctant to pull away from the social media drama to join the family at dinner for actual conversation. Having family members wiggly at the table because they're eager to return to their devices for fear of missing out on something is common.

Less Social Interaction

Time alone without interacting with others can be a lonely endeavor. People do need people.

Depression

And of course, spending too much time in isolation can lead to depressed moods. Detaching from others isn't natural. One way to work through this is to video chat with others, or if open, spend time in a local restaurant, or coffee shop where you can "plug in" and still be around the hustle and bustle of people. Outside venues are often available where the virus fears prevail.

No matter where you turn or in what part of the world you reside, somehow you are impacted by COVID-19. We've moved into a new reality—at least for the time being—which will dictate how we live our lives and perhaps how we view the aging process. Some will take a step back to normalcy, embracing life and all it offers while putting less attention on the façade, or outer exterior of the body.

Shopping For Essentials

In the early days of the coronavirus, I stayed home when not working. I recall finally making my way to Sam's Club to pick up essentials, as I'd not done any shopping—real shopping—in almost three weeks, due to the pandemic. "Essentials" has become the buzzword in our COVID society, moving from "primping" to look your best, to the survival mode of buying food. All of the cosmetic counters, dermatologist, and cosmetic surgeries were put on hold as the pandemic took front place, and *essential* no longer meant having manicures and pedicures, haircuts, or eyebrows tweezed, let alone full eyelifts.

Going to the grocery was daunting for sure. My mask and disposable latex-free gloves donned, *our new norm*, I made my way through the aisles, conscious of keeping my distance by at least six feet from the other shoppers. I used the scan-and-go feature on my phone to avoid the line and the cashier, fumbling all the while, with my gloves adding more challenges to my scan than hoped-for. But shop I did, through the maze of challenges, with my face mask slipping, sweating, as it's hot to wear, but so thankful to have one.

My phone dropped out two to three times as I awkwardly continued, with my synthetic gloves getting caught in the keys. My phone didn't read my face, either, but instead required me to punch the numbers. I quickly learned the phone couldn't scan my face with a mask—I looked different to the device.

While we cycled through these different emotions of denial and acceptance, I couldn't help but think about Kubler-Ross as I bargained while coming to grips with this "new" normal. Early in my undergraduate years, I learned about Elizabeth

Kubler-Ross, a Swiss-American psychiatrist, who in her 1969 book entitled, *On Death and Dying: What the Dying Have to Teach Doctors, Nurses, Clergy, and Their Own Families,* presented the five stages of grief, also known as the Kubler-Ross model.

Though originally this model was patterned on grief stages of the dying, it morphed into a representation plugged into many scenarios of grief and loss. The five stages chronologically are: denial, anger, bargaining, depression, and acceptance. We started off hard-pressed to believe (*denial*) such a pandemic was really going on—but it was—yet the day was gorgeous, the sun was out, and the sky was a piercing blue, laced with chunks of white clouds. We power forth (*acceptance*).

Everything seemed to be okay—but we knew it wasn't. We had that gnawing deep inside that someone somewhere was taking a last breath—and possibly that person was someone we knew. Life can be a challenge for many plagued by the inner chatter and self-bashing about not being pretty enough or young enough, but with this pandemic, we had a tough time of a different sort—how could we cycle through this?

For many, *depression* took hold alongside this forced isolation and social distancing. But then we *bargained* that if we wore the mask and gloves when we went out for essentials and stayed inside at home the remaining time, then soon, soon we could return to normal. And for others, *denial* was firmly in place as they congregated in large groups as if nothing was going on, as if people weren't dying and ventilators weren't in demand for those who couldn't breathe on their own. Some cycled to *anger*, mad that this invisible thing was interrupting our normalcy.

My trip to Sam's was usually a 40-minute drive — but on this trip, the streets were bare — I made it in less than twenty minutes. Not a lot of cars were on the road, and few stores were open. Most of those driving by were going home, not meandering unless absolutely necessary and essential — that word again. Peeking over at the car next to me, eyes met mine — their faces were covered too.

The feeling through all this has been almost as if we were dream-walking through our nearly familiar world, but we weren't; this was reality — all this was really happening. And regardless of whether we were introvert types or extraverts, this seemed ominous at best. The restaurants were closed, the bars were closed, and even with much resistance, the casinos were the last to shut down.

Churches, synagogues, and temples closed — yet liquor stores remained open to prevent the alcoholic from full-blown withdrawal. Though understandable and an important preventative measure, that provision blew my mind. Prayer and congregating for both extrovert and classic isolator was now removed.

My husband, though at retirement age, is a typical workaholic with no intention to slow down. Now, for the first time in all of his adult life, he was stuck at home, creating chores around the house to keep busy and productive, while I worked remotely alone from the office. As a natural introvert I've been okay—sort of—but I also feel disconnected from the goings on in the outside world. My husband, a natural extrovert, has been not so okay as he's been yearning for people and conversation with his once-bustling restaurant now forced closed.

So in a daze, my mind wandering in disbelief, I continued to wait in line four blocks away from Sam's Club—trying to maintain the six-foot rule to the best of my ability. The woman behind me, chatting in Spanish about the crisis to a loved one I assumed was far away, was inching up on me, no doubt without realization. Slowly we made our way to the front of the line and into the store.

Some people used panic buying online or at the grocery stores to cope with their fear—you know the ones, hoarding toilet paper—but I planned to make a beeline right to *that* very aisle as the thought of running out of the precious white puffy stuff *was* terrifying. I'm human—and I panic, too.

I still had access to Facebook and the different social medias to connect with family and friends. And my sisters and I were all bonding in our group text—reminiscing about the good ole days when not so long ago we were on the west coast of Florida hanging out, as four sisters will. We had a week of walking, facials, and feeling spry and youthful for our ages—a sixty-something foursome.

Living in South Florida, I have been in quite a hotspot, even now as I write and edit, and my dear friends are in New York (much recovered from being the hotspot early on) and my family in Chicago (a city not doing overly well)—with really no escape for anybody. Seems the circumstances indicate the virus is running hard with just a matter of time before it affects everyone—if it hasn't already. And of course this increases the panic—making home a safe zone— more isolation for the introvert a condition quite painful for the extrovert. But staying at home has provided great practice for those of us nearing retirement. Perhaps we've had an opportunity to learn what is beneficial in filling our days, and what isn't.

Perhaps we all needed a reset, a time to start journaling, to clean out the garage or closet—perhaps you've held onto lovely clothes that you no longer wear, and someone else could use. My husband, the extrovert, painted doors, completely cleaned and painted our vanity, and deep-cleaned spots in our home we've not looked at in a while. Even our robot vacuum, which we fondly call Burt, made his way through the garage, snatching up this and that from the floor.

Home once again with my stash of essentials, I entered into Easter weekend, watching Mass on television, eating a simple meal, video chatting with our son and daughter-in law—though they live only minutes away. Isolation and introversion were forced on us...a new norm.

But regardless of whether we're introverts or extroverts, or possibly a combination of the two, we still need to be who we are by living exactly as we are.

Perhaps, indeed, this is a time to reset, as you'll see in Chapter 10.

Personal Inventory Questions

1. *If I am not for myself, who will be for me?* We do need to start with the personal self to be our best self in order to help others. *Yet, if I am for myself alone, of what good am I?* How does this line of thinking impact you?

2. Spending too much time in isolation can lead to depressed moods. Detaching from others isn't natural. One way to work through this is to video chat with others, or if open, spend time in a local restaurant, or coffee shop to "plug in" and still be around the hustle and bustle of people. Have you found that isolation led to depression for you? What have you done to combat this.

3. What are you—an introvert or an extrovert? Do you tend to be a loner? Or do you tend to be social? Are you a little bit of both? How does that work?

4. During the first part of the pandemic of COVID-19, did you let go of your primping and pampering and isolate? How did this impact you in terms of your aging process? Did you forget about issues of aging and turn to an obsession over fears of the virus?

5. How would you define yourself in the circle of yin and yang? The introvert and extrovert dance between the yin and yang of opposite forces, which are seen as interconnected and

counterbalancing. Where do you dance? What does your dance tell you about you?

6. The obsession over aging begins to take a back seat as the fear of a real issue, such as the coronavirus, takes the front seat. What aging concerns popped up for you during the pandemic?

7. One post that imprinted in my mind was passed around at LivingChristian.org: *While you wash your hands, PRAY for 20 seconds. Let's change the world!* Can you imagine if everyone really did pray for 20 seconds, how many prayers would be sent out into the ether — the heavens? Did you find you began to move closer to the God of your understanding during the pandemic? Did you move away?

8. The Kubler-Ross model originally was patterned after the grief stages of the dying; it morphed into a representation that is plugged into many scenarios of grief and loss. The five stages chronologically are: denial, anger, bargaining, depression, and acceptance. Where did and do you fit in this model during troubling times?

9. The feeling we've had is almost as if we were dream-walking through the pandemic but we weren't. The virus was reality — it really happened. And regardless of whether you're an introvert type or an extrovert, the sense we have of this is an ominous one, at best. Have you felt a split from reality at times?

10. Some people during the pandemic used panic buying online or at the grocery stores to cope — you know the ones, hoarding toilet paper. Did you hoard TP? Did you find yourself hoarding any products? What about hair dye or something to help you to feel youthful?

Chapter 10

A Time to Reset

And now here is my secret,
a very simple secret:
It is only with the heart
that one can see rightly;
What is essential is invisible to the eye.
~Antoine de Saint-Exupery

"What is essential is invisible to the eye." I never knew this to be so true as when we went through the shutdown with the coronavirus. Everything seemed to go into slow motion. Everything in our world shut down. My office emptied, stores closed, my husband closed his restaurant of 35 years. And all the "essentials" that we had come to depend on seemed to become "nonessential."

FALL IN *love* WITH BOOKS

I ♥ READING

H10491 (13667930) upstartpromotions.com
© 1999, 2010 James Dean

We had a choice to kick and scream, but of course that wouldn't stop what was about to unfold. Instead, many chose to lean into it — to regroup and do a reset.

And in that stillness, miracles began to unfold — as it is *only with the heart that one can see rightly*. But you can't see rightly if you're running and pushing for the next something.

The shutdown was a raw awakening for many of us, as all our pampering we took for granted came to a total stop. So much we relied on fit into the "nonessential" category. And hospitals, nurses, police, and doctors were part of the "essential" group. Not only were we social distancing and staying in our homes, with the exception of work for those of us declared essential, but also all nonessential stores and businesses shut down.

And with that, my massage therapist, hair salon, manicurist, and pedicurist, along with the dermatologist, dental hygienist, and esthetician all closed. The primping and fixing-up stopped completely. And this was not only for me, but also for all of us, everywhere. I began to see gray in my hair I'd never seen before. Sure, it was there, but if you highlight and dye your roots all the time, you really don't know the gray is present. At first, I thought the color was kind of pretty, but as my hair grew longer and longer, I questioned exactly how pretty it was.

The appointments for all my primping would have taken place during the first week of the shutdown, so by week 16 I could see the changes really take hold. And not just for me, but also for the newscasters, patients I worked with on video sessions, neighbors, Facebook friends — all of us, with the exception of those who had people sneak in so they could have some of these things done. Most of us looked as though we could use a "touch up" of some sort. As time marched on, I began to appreciate, *really appreciate,* those who went along with the state we were in — living exactly as they were (at least for now)...and tapping into a reset.

So what is involved in a reset? Does that mean not to dye your hair or have your teeth cleaned or polish your nails? Absolutely not. But when these luxuries are taken away, we have time to reflect on who we are in the naked, original form, and what is important to us. We're forced to slow down and enter into the stillness of life.

A Tweet to Action

I have many friends on Twitter, and one of them, Ian, from across the pond, wrote about his depression and Lyme disease and how he was an "at risk" person and needed to stay at home. He was on week 10 of his self-isolation. He feared his depression would spiral out of control, so he took charge of his situation and began to work on the novel he'd tossed to the side months before.

Ian dusted himself off along with his novel, and began to write again. To his glee, he not only finished his novel, adding 300,000 words, completing his trilogy, he also warded off his depression. He did a reset and made it work, taking on a lemonade-out-of-lemons attitude.

Ian is VERY social, a walking his neighborhood, visiting the neighbors, walking around the park, and hanging out with his friends daily kind of social. When he sank to his lows after his diagnosis with Lyme disease, he pushed away friends, and sank lower. But soon after therapy, he began to climb out of his dark hole, though next, with the mandatory shut-in allowing only one outdoor walk daily, he feared a decline. Then Ian took action and reset to his own benefit. You can too.

One particular morning I was having a frustrating time. Alexa wouldn't tell me the daily news brief because she was on the fritz; my big toe on my right foot was hurting because my nails need trimming and an ingrown toenail was trying to take over; and on top of that, the daily Mass I like to tune into from St. Patrick's Cathedral in New York wasn't behaving on Sirius Radio. Argggg. The morning wasn't going well.

But as life would have it, something better was waiting for me. So since Sirius wasn't behaving, I then turned to a podcast because I wanted or *needed* something to listen to—but before I could make my choice, all of a sudden, Oprah started talking. I guess the decision was made for me. Oprah was talking to Dr. Alan Lightman about "How to Lead a Less Hurried Life" on her Super Soul Series.

The podcast was a very short 18-minute talk with an amazing punch. The discussion concerned rushing to do this and that, and missing the moment right in front of us. Dr. Lightman spoke about slowing down. He discussed connecting to the universe, the earth, and the animals. He talked about moving away from the busyness and seeing what's right here in the now.

I didn't need the podcast to teach me to live in the now, as I've always known and prided myself on living in the present, making this my best practice — but somehow, between writing books, working my practice, writing blogs, and connecting to social media to bond "out there," I became caught up in work. I missed out on the life in front of me — and I didn't even know it. *Life marches on and waits for nobody.*

Ian, entering his latter sixties, learned this lesson when he sank into his dark depression for two decades. Like many of us, he began regrouping and resetting with a forced shut-in — fearing he'd sink into the darkness of despair. I know this to be true with my patients, who are also shut in. Many, like Ian, with serious illnesses, making them vulnerable to this virus, were forced to stay in and social distance, even more than others.

If I've learned one good thing from the terrible pandemic, it's that I've been working too many hours, letting life pass me by. I've slowed down working now, not wanting to be alone in the office late in the evening, and because of that, I'm spending more time with my husband and pets. I'm home these days when it's still light out, permitting a bike ride; dinner with my husband; and watching my dog, Gracie, play in the yard; or maybe I even take the time to enjoy a night swim—all things I missed working long and late hours.

The short Oprah podcast was chock full of words I really had to hear. I was guilty of rushing round and not taking it easy. I knew the truth deep inside, but I needed the podcast to nudge me into realizing the time had come for a reset. Perhaps you need a reset too. And what I realized is it doesn't matter what age we are for our reset. And I learned that connecting to our spiritual self often happens when we least expect it.

Dr. Lightman described his spiritual awakening when he was returning to an island after midnight, alone in his boat on the ocean. He lay down in his boat and looked up at the sky and felt as if he were falling into infinity—as though he were merging with the stars…the cosmos…part of something larger than himself, feeling a connection to the spiritual realm. This was a personal experience, an un-provable but real connection to all living things in the universe. It was his spiritual awakening.

Oprah, too, described her awakening when walking with a friend and the sky looked like a painting with a sliver of the moon hung in such a way with the clouds hanging low, that it brought her a feeling of great awe.

I, too, have had my spiritual moments, the biggest being giving birth to my son, Benjamin, which I wrote about in my first book, *Release Your Obsession with Food: Heal from the Inside Out*. I moved out of my body and up above "myself," to look down and watch the entire birthing. I wasn't on any medicine or epidurals. This was simply a totally natural, painless birthing experience. It was my spiritual awakening.

Dr. Alan Lightman, an MIT professor of humanities, a physicist, and a bestselling author, talked about how he also embraced spirituality. The idea of a scientist embracing spirituality caught my attention—and Oprah's too. An article he'd written that was published in *The Atlantic*, introduced Oprah to his work. The article was entitled "The Virus Is a Reminder of Something Lost Long Ago."

The Atlantic was founded in 1857 in Boston, Massachusetts, as *The Atlantic Monthly*. It's a literary and cultural commentary magazine that from the start published leading writers' commentary on the abolition of slavery, education, and other major issues in contemporary political affairs. And this very article was what intrigued Oprah enough to interview Dr. Lightman, and I'm glad she did, as it was perfect for me to listen to that morning.

I pressed on to hear the professor's message as to how he thought the COVID-19 pandemic offered us an opportunity to lead less hurried lives. That morning, prior to listening in, I'd started my daily morning walk with my jaw clenched really tight, I was angry that my day had begun with nothing going my way, and now here was this guy talking about slowing down. And I did. I recognized I'd fallen into an angry pattern, resenting what I couldn't control— the virus and our new norm.

As Dr. Lightman and Oprah talked, I began to take notice of my surroundings, surroundings I see every single day — but on this day I *really* took note. I observed the lovely red hibiscus bushes blooming in full fanfare, with yellow butterflies hovering and fluttering, drunken with the scent. The palm trees were swaying against an amazing blue sky, and sailboats were filling Southlake, which runs into the Intercoastal and Atlantic Ocean.

One sailboat in particular had caught my attention over weeks and weeks that had turned into months and months. It was abandoned, I presumed. It was a deep-black boat with a dark-red trim around the base, a white interior with a spinning star propped up on the sail, a dove at the helm. The vessel was quite old, but handsome for sure. I watched and watched, days, weeks, and months for signs of life on that boat — but nothing. NO person on board.

And I imagined what jumping on that boat and sailing away and writing to my heart's content would be like. I wanted to run away from the virus and all that it brings. I yearned for a restart, so to speak, to sail away from COVID-19, from the news, from the jobs lost, from the deaths, from the sicknesses — just sail away.

And now as Dr. Lightman spoke of stillness and how it's so important to our daily lives, and that our country now has a chance to nurture what he calls the "inner self," I began to calm down. I began to feel better. I began to realize somehow I'd lost my balance and needed to reset in order to embrace life exactly as it was now.

The parrots were out in full bloom that morning as they feasted on a birdhouse filled with luscious seed an owner puts out for them every few days. And this day was extra special as blue jays, red cardinals, and parrots of all sorts were waiting for their turn to nibble the seed mixture, as were doves, squirrels, and sparrows. All in unity, all taking turns. I felt one with the animals, earth, and sky.

At some point, Oprah said, "We are all here getting a reset," and my ears perked up, as this was the same thing I'd been saying to my patients for weeks now. The words were resonating, as they were familiar, but I hadn't been listening for myself. I seemed to have felt I needed permission that I too could reset. And maybe you also are looking for permission to reset, especially if you're turning the corner in the aging process. Is it possible to reset at a certain age or are we simply set?

We do have to slow down as a society and as individuals, and the fact that a worldwide pandemic came along to wake us up is pretty amazing. That we need to choose a less hurried life was Dr. Lightman's message, and I listened and embraced what he had to say. Prior to this shutdown and slowdown, I was enmeshed in my work, writing in the morning and evening, seeing ten patients in-between, walking five miles in the morning, and reading somewhere in all of that.

My life was harried. I'd get up with the first sign of light, walk five miles, eat breakfast, prepare for work, write for an hour, and then hit it at work until 9 in the evening, returning home super late, only to spend a few hours feeding Oliver my parrot and giving him some time out of his cage. Then I'd play with Gracie, then write, and with the last bits of my time check in on my husband and his day.

But now, after the shutdown, I took a step back and realized all the primping and fussing and rushing weren't me living exactly as I am but rather chasing and gobbling minutes of precious life rather than embracing. Are you doing that too?

Dr. Lightman attracted my attention so much that I purchased his book, *In Praise of Wasting Time*, to devour more of his message, to slow down. He speaks of the digital grid, which "...replaces in-the-flesh reality with virtual reality, and that virtual reality is loud, all consuming, dehumanizing and relentless. It can crowd out the rest of life. And it rushes ahead, without waiting for anyone."

So true! Now interestingly, this very book you're reading is a book on releasing your obsession with aging, so you'd think with this forced slowdown, we'd all have plenty of time to reset and become still. But do we?

A Reset at Any Age

My sister Debbie is not a fan of the digital world. She would much rather have the human touch versus texting, a fact that she vocalizes every chance she can.

She loves long visits on the phone and in person whenever possible. And of course, in my busy life, I don't have hours to lavish on the phone, unless I'm multi-tasking, like walking and talking during my morning promenade. And we live states apart, so seeing one another in person is a rare treat.

Debbie is retired, as is her husband. They chose to retire young and live the good life. And they do. They're busy and productive in their own right. My husband and I aren't retired. Though the shutdown forced my husband to be in "retirement" mode, this manner of operation is not feeling too swift for him. With this forced pause, we have an opportunity to take a step back and reset, regroup, and strategize how we want our years to unfold from now going forward. But something stirs within both of us that we're not working to our full capacity with the forced inactivity.

But isn't that the message, to become still, embrace the quiet, and connect? Maybe we can find a means to connect in a human way but still be productive—yet not in a hamster-on-a-wheel kind of way. My sister Debbie purchased our mother's farmhouse with a ginormous barn and acreage, and is having the time of her life making it beautiful, doing most of the work herself. The house sits on plush forestry land with nature in the palm of her hand. Now that's embracing retirement in a productive sort of way. That's a reset to me, not a step back.

We experience different stages in our lives, such as working our way through the formative years and schooling, entering college, being married and having babies, followed by the empty nest period, to retirement. We race from one milestone to the next, not knowing where we'll become stuck, and which parts we'll sail through. My patients in their later years seem to still live life with the same urgency as the younger patients, but aging is at the forefront of their minds.

One weekend, I escaped to our getaway home with Oliver (my eclectic parrot) and Gracie (my Swiss shepherd) without my husband—as he thought he'd open his restaurant with Phase II on to bring our state back after the shutdown. Sadly, he was stopped before opening because of legalities and paperwork that needed to be in place for liability, just in case somebody contracted the coronavirus. (Of course, who knows where one might pick it up as opportunities abound, but that's another story.)

So here I was writing about resetting, standing still, and slowing down, and I received a text from my husband: "Good morning, another sleepless night dreaming and dreaming. It's funny how the mind works. I went to bed early, was up at 4:00 a.m. again for at least one hour, maybe more. In my dreams, I was working at the café and playing music for a large crowd. I was very young, which is a good thing." He went on to say a few romantic things that I'll save just for us.

Many of us have the feeling that something needs to be done. Maybe innately within us is to *do* at all times. My husband is a musician who plays on weekends and runs his café daily without taking days off. He loves the rush of both jobs. He's social, *very* social, unlike me, who prefers the alone time, the quiet. The virus and shutdown forced him to stop working. Just stop and be, something he hadn't done before.

Perhaps kicking back and slowing down and dancing to our own beat is okay. We have no reason to fret over time, weather, or that feeling we're missing out on something. Maybe we can sit still and let the happenings happen—in their own time, at their own beat. But for many of us this isn't so easy, especially when the relaxed pace is forced. We're all works in progress, and all like to control our own outcomes. Then sometimes God has a different plan, and we simply have to go with it. Not so simple for many.

Though both my husband and I are at retirement age, we aren't the retiring types. We love our work; it gives us the juice to get up each day. My husband's famous words always have been, "Retire? Retire to what?" And I agree. We'll both continue to feed our creative sides, me with my writing, and he with music, while I work with patients and he feeds the community at his restaurant.

Those I speak to who are now retired admit they're not competing with work, but are still competing with the clock, and competing with the self. Sandy, referencing her retired life, says, "When we worked, we had to fit into work clothes, put on makeup, you know, *had* to look good. We can still look good, but in the reset mode, we can stop competing with others, and just be."

A time to reset — a time to renew — is sometimes forced on us, and sometimes we gracefully find it.

But listen to this secret, Antoine de Saint-Exupery's secret: "And now here is my secret, a very simple secret: it is only with the heart that one can see rightly; what is essential is invisible to the eye." What is essential is invisible to the eye, and I never knew this to be so true as when we went through the shutdown with the coronavirus.

That period seemed as if everything went into slow motion. Everything shut down. Life isn't about how much work we do or how much money we have or how young we are. What makes a life, a person, is what lies within — that only with the heart one can see rightly. What is truly essential is invisible to the eye. Wise words as we move into the matter of, age does not define you (Chapter 11).

Personal Inventory Questions

1. What is essential is invisible to the eye, and I never knew this to be so true as when we went through the shutdown with the coronavirus. This period seemed as if everything went into slow motion. Everything shut down. I know it shut down for you too. Did you welcome the stillness? Did you fight it, or go with it?
2. The primping and fixing-up stopped as the shut-in ensued. And this was not only for me, but also for all of us, everywhere. What physical changes did

you notice? How did it impact you? Did you feel frumpy or welcome the change?

3. Ian, from across the pond, tweeted about his depression and Lyme disease, and how he was an "at risk" person and needed to self-isolate. On week ten in isolation, fearing his depression would spiral out of control, he took charge of his situation and began to work on the novel he'd tossed aside months before. What project did you dust off and start to work on? Or did you clean out a closet perhaps? How did this impact your reset?

4. One particular morning I was feeling frustrated. But I tuned into a podcast that was meaningful and something I needed to hear. Has this ever happened to you? I'm sure it did. Search your mind for when and how a surprising lesson had an impact on you.

5. We do have to slow down, and the fact that a worldwide pandemic had to occur to wake us up is pretty amazing. Choose a less hurried life was Dr. Lightman's podcast message that I listened to and embraced. What message did you embrace during the pandemic?

6. If I've learned one good thing from the terrible pandemic it's that I've been working too many hours, letting life pass me by. What have you learned by slowing down? Did you slow down?

7. Miracles happen all the time, but sometimes we're not paying attention, and the busyness of life blocks the miraculous from our view. What

spiritual awakening or miracle have you experienced?

8. The patients I work with in their later years seem to still live life with the same urgency as my younger patients, but aging is at the forefront of their thoughts. Is it at the forefront of your thoughts? Does it change the urgency in which you live life?

9. My sister Debbie is retired, as is her husband. They chose to retire young and live the good life. They're busy and productive in their own right. Do you wish to retire? If so, what does retirement look like to you?

10. Perhaps kicking back and slowing down and dancing to your own beat is okay. We have no reason to fret over time, weather, or that feeling we're missing out on something. Why not make a list of your reset as you stand still and watch the miracles unfold.

Chapter 11

Age Does Not Define You

Begin with the end in mind.
~Stephen Covey

By the time you arrive at this chapter, you'll have a hint that age doesn't define you — or at least that's the message I hope to impart from the start. And to begin with the conclusion in mind is a perfect representation of this entire book. We should think about what lies ahead from the beginning, as well as what we might expect all along our ramble.

How do you want to live your life? Remember, how we spend our days is how we live our lives, as mentioned in an earlier chapter, and now we might consider how we want to continue, keeping the end, the last stage of life, in mind.

NOT

You are not your age,
nor the size of clothes you wear.
You are not a weight.
Or the color of your hair.
You are not your name,
or the dimples in your cheeks.
You are all the books you read,
and all the words you speak.
You are your croaky morning voice,
and the smiles you try to hide,
You're the sweetness in your laughter
and every tear you've cried.
You're the songs you sing so loudly,
when you know you're all alone.
You're the places that you've been to,
and the one that you call home.
You're the things that you believe in,
and the people that you love.
You're the photos in your bedroom,
and the future you dream of.
You're made of so much beauty,
but it seems that you forgot.
When you decided that you were defined,
by all the things you're not.
~Erin Hansen

This is a brilliant piece I happened upon, written by Erin Hansen, at the time nineteen years old, a girl wise beyond her years. She writes for me, she writes for you, she writes for the young, and she writes for the old. Stumbling upon this piece was no accident— finding it as I wrote this book was meant to be.

We are our experiences. We are our laughter and smiles. The lines on our faces show how we lived out our experiences through laughter, smiles, and tears. We're not our age; hence, age does not define us. Surely we may slow down and have a kink here and there, but age is a number—and we have a choice how we'll spend those numbers. Imagine your nineties now; how do you want to feel?

When Depression Peeks Through

Depression may find its way as your mind and body go through changes. You may happen upon some sad days or days when you wish for the past, a time you were young and more energetic—this is normal. How you move beyond your down days is key to how you embrace the inevitable changes.

Gregory L. Jantz, PhD, in his *Moving Beyond Depression: A Whole-Person Approach to Healing*, writes: "The pace of life can exhaust us. The patterns of life can undercut us. Unexpected dilemmas, such as the loss of a job, the illness or death of a loved one, a financial crisis, the necessity of a move, or personal health problems can erode our emotional equilibrium."

Life will present unpredictable ups and downs that can knock us to our knees. Though such times can be rough, these very experiences are part of what we build our lifelong memories on. These very events give us strength and carve out who we are—but our age isn't the thing that molds us. We have experiences from our first spark of existence back in the womb, all the way to the end. Those are what make us who we are.

Fear of aging often stems from much we've had to bear in life watching what others have undergone or suffered through. When we experience a significant loss, depression can occur. Going though life's events shapes what we think life will be. We may think we understand what follows, before we enter the next phase, but our view is skewed, most often deviates from the actual happening.

For sure we all will feel sad or depressed at different times in our lives. Feeling our mood slip downward is normal—a reaction to loss or life's inevitable struggles. But when intense sadness persists, including feeling helpless, hopeless, and worthless, and these emotions last for many days to weeks, months, or even years and prevent us from living a quality life, the condition may be something more than just sadness.

As we age, the fear of not having independence, or losing our mobility or thought process can be gripping, but the imagined situation isn't slated to necessarily come about, as surely we know and observe many clear-minded, self-reliant, happy older persons — maybe even more than we see young teens in such a state.

The epidemic of depression, anxiety, and suicide is a real problem taking hold of the hearts and souls of our younger population. Often, the severity of such a state goes undetected as the young person struggles to find their footing in adult life. The depression could be situational, based on the circumstances — and that's true for both young and older persons.

Clinical depression is a treatable medical condition. Patients who come to me with depression most often have a depression based on something they endured that became so unbearable they needed help from a professional. The *Diagnostic and Statistical Manual of Mental Disorders, Fifth Edition* (*DSM-5, 2013*), the most recent manual clinicians and doctors look at to evaluate mental disorders, is used as a gauge and diagnosing tool. According to the DSM-5 from the American Psychiatric Association, you have depression when you have five or more of the following symptoms for at least two weeks:

- You have a depressed mood during most of the day, especially in the morning.
- You feel tired or lack energy almost every day.
- You feel worthless or guilty almost every day.
- You have a hard time focusing, remembering details, and making decisions.
- You can't sleep or you sleep too much almost every day.

- You have almost no interest or pleasure in most activities nearly every day.
- You think often about death or suicide (not just a fear of death).
- You feel restless or slowed down.
- You've lost or gained weight.

You may also:

- Feel irritable and restless.
- Lose pleasure in life.
- Overeat or stop feeling hungry.
- Have aches or pains, headaches, cramps, or digestive problems that don't go away or resolve with treatment.
- Have sad, anxious, or "empty" feelings.

This list is by no means a diagnosis of you, the reader, but discussing depression is necessary when considering aging or the fear of aging. When you let age define you, it can bring forth a host of feelings and expectations from examples of age you witnessed growing up that may make you fearful. Your little antennae are not quite developed at a young age, and you may have misunderstood what you thought was happening.

What you've seen may not be a true reading of what aging is, especially in a time such as ours when young is in, and old is out. When people search high and low for products to retain their youth, and various approaches aren't working, or they themselves are starting to decline, depression can ensue.

Keep in mind the listing from the DSM-5 is a list of symptoms that a person suffering from depression *might* have. Indicators aren't going to be the same exact ones for everyone.

Begin With the End in Mind

But wouldn't life be easier if in the cozy womb we began with the end in mind. If we knew exactly where we were headed on our life journey before we even began. If we knew all the twists and turns that were coming, so we could dodge the heartaches and painful days that await us—as surely they do.

Beginning with the end in mind would be great, but most of us don't. Some people already know exactly what their careers will be when they're young children. They just know. But that's not the norm. Most of us change our minds many times before landing on what we'll do for a living and what kind of mates we'll share our lives with. But, many do seem to know what they're aiming for early in the game of life.

When Benjamin, my youngest son, was little, he spoke of being a fisherman when he grew up. I recall saying, "Great, you could own a fleet of boats and fish for everyone." He didn't grow up to be a fisherman, but his friend who dreamed of being a doctor when they were kids actually did become a doctor.

Ironically, that same son of ours, who resented and was adamant in opposing the idea of being an attorney, which we always said he should become because he had the gift of arguing eloquently, wanted no part of it—and then became exactly that. So, we don't always know where the road will take us, but if we did, would life be simpler? Would ageing be less taxing and reduce the fear of growing up and growing old?

If you knew you were going to write that great novel, or marry the love of your life, or bear amazing, loving children who grow up kind and caring, living their best life, would knowing that ending make a difference at the start? Yes, this is something to consider deeply. Though I can't help but wonder if we knew how our lives would unfold before they unfolded, would we lose the mystery, the magic, and excitement of the unknown?

When my first marriage ended with betrayal and abandonment, breaking my heart in two, I had no idea my true-life partner was out there, waiting for me. Had I known, would the knowledge have lessened the pain? Should we lessen the pain? Perhaps no, because we wouldn't learn life's lessons if we always knew the outcome.

But if we believed in something greater, something grander, and the faith in that belief carried us through, we might be able to navigate through the years with more ease—fearless.

If Only My Nose Were Turned Up

A while back I had a session with a thirteen-year-old we'll call Cassandra, who began restricting her food and purging anything she ate by way of reckless exercising throughout the night—100 jumping jacks,

191

100 crunches, 100 leg lifts—on and on until she felt she'd burned through the calories. She was fixated on her size—but not because she wanted to become skinny for her body, but rather for her face.

I wondered what sparked this behavior, only to learn Cassandra didn't like her face. As we dug deeper, she reported that a child in second grade told her she had a fat face. And since then, the thought of her *distorted* face possessed her. It wasn't shaped right—according to her.

Cassandra went on to say that her face didn't look thin enough, but if she sucked the air out of them, and stopped eating, *it was perfect.* She went on to say, "Ever since I was little, my face was fat, and I feared wrinkles." Wrinkles! How could a little child think about wrinkles?

So this girl, who had, by the way, a beautiful face, believed she needed sunken-in cheeks and practiced sucking them in every chance she could, resembling a goldfish with wide eyes as she leaned into the screen during the video chat to look closer at herself not realizing I too could see her moving into and staring at herself on the screen.

I saw this many times with many patients over the video sessions, all scrutinizing themselves—looking for flaws of some sort. Cassandra practiced this behavior so much that it became her new norm. At first I thought what she did was a tick of some sort, not a trained behavior. When she didn't resemble a fish with her sucked-in cheeks, she was stunning in every way.

I understood where Cassandra was coming from, as when I was young, I had an issue with my nose that I've written about in previous books. I was convinced my nose was humungous — to the point I'd sit with my finger propped right under my nose in the hope of forcing it to tip upward. You know, those cute little ski-jump noses that turn upward. My nose is strong — when I was a kid, one man described it as a Roman nose — which didn't help stop my obsession with propping it up every chance I got.

So this young girl also had an obsession, but hers amounted to the desire to stay young forever. Aging, she decided, meant you couldn't do the fun things you did as a kid. She went on to say, "Aging means you're crippled and old. Aging means life no longer is enjoyable because you have to work and do grown-up things. Laughter is snuffed out and smiles nonexistent." She longed for simpler times when her parents were loving and embracing, when family was whole, and the world felt right. She wanted Christmas as her normal.

When parents dissolve their marriage, divorce takes a toll on kids in different ways. My experience was similar to that of this young girl in that I was stripped of normalcy on every level when Mom whisked her six kids to a remote town where we lived in our non-winterized cottage with promises of how much *fun* we were going to have living where we summered.

Life there wasn't fun. The winters were cold and long. The town was critical of outsiders, so I never felt

I belonged. My siblings quickly dispersed into the real grownup world, leaving me behind. I grew up fast and furious. And my fear of adulthood blossomed and life there ignited my eating disorder.

Age does not define us nor does depression—our mere existence and how we spend our days defines us. If we focus on the end in the beginning, we can have a roadmap for how we wish to live. In living our authentic lives (Chapter 8), we touch on living our bliss, which should be what defines us, not age. And now we move on to eating disorders and aging in Chapter 12.

Personal Inventory Questions

1. What does "begin with the end in mind" mean to you? What would life look like if you knew what would happen before you started?
2. When I stumbled across Erin Hansen's poem *Not,* I was thrilled to find her wise words. I was searching for something to express the thought that age doesn't define us. Surely this nineteen-year-old seemed to grasp that at an early age. How did her poem affect you?
3. We are our experiences. We are our laughter and smiles. The lines on our faces show how we lived our experiences through laughter, smiles, and tears. We are not our age; hence, age doesn't define us. Do you agree?
4. Gregory L. Jantz, PhD, in *Moving Beyond Depression: A Whole-Person Approach to Healing*

states, "The pace of life can exhaust us." Does it exhaust you? Would you slow down if you could?

5. Fear of aging often stems from what we endured in early life by watching what others have undergone or suffered through. What is your understanding of aging? Who did you get this idea from? Trace back as far as you can to determine where your understanding of aging stems from.

6. When intense sadness continues, including feeling helpless, hopeless, and worthless, and it lasts for many days to weeks or longer and prevents you from living a quality life, you may have something more than sadness. Have you ever experienced this emotional rut? Are you experiencing it now? What changes could you implement to move out of this persistent feeling?

7. Beginning with the end in mind would be great but most of us don't. Some people know exactly what their career will be later in life when they're still young children. Did you know? Or, did your parents or a person of authority suggest what you *should* be when you grew up?

8. As we age, the fear of not having our independence or losing our mobility or thought process can be gripping, but this doesn't necessarily lie ahead. Surely we know many clear-minded, self-reliant, happy older persons — maybe even more than teens with such attributes. Is the possibility of deterioration one of your fears? How

can you change that fear to a powerful insight about a possible positive future?

9. Did you fear wrinkles or aging as a young child like the girl I described? Did you do something to change that fear, or does it still haunt you?

10. Often we become hung up on a body part when we're very young. The fixation could be because someone made a remark to you, and it imbedded in your thoughts, taking control. For me, the comment was about my *Roman* nose, and for the young girl described, the statement was that her face was too full. What was the turning point for you?

Chapter 12

Eating Disorders and Aging

Come to the edge.
We can't.
We're afraid.
We can't.
We will fall!
Come to the edge.
And they came.
And he pushed them.
And they flew.
~Guillaume Apollinaire

People are terrified of falling...Period. The first time I ever rode a bicycle without the training wheels, I was beyond terrified. I was immobilized. I was frozen in place. And then at some point, I pedaled and pedaled, and the bike just kept going. I got it! Or the first time I swam out to the raft as a kid at Silver Lake in Wautoma, Wisconsin. I was very afraid—the dark, deep water was more than frightening—I thought it would swallow me, and it didn't. We *can* fly—you and me.

We can fly, and we can move past change, and blossom. Where is the fear of change coming from? Take a step back and look at the origination of the fear. Where did we first become stuck? In my case, and that of most of my patient load, and possibly you, the reader, our discomfort started with the fear of not being in control as life began to change—way back, when we were tiny, little people. And from this despair, many of us were caught in the fear of our body changes, wanting to be thin, strong, and muscular. Perhaps we thought we could regulate our bodies in some way when we couldn't manage life's many challenges.

And during the aging process, that same fear of losing control lurks. Often our obsessions spring forth because of the road less traveled—the unknown. And that same angst over taking the leap and falling arises, with us not realizing we can soar to amazing heights. But instead, the unknown and "what ifs" loom so large and petrifying in our minds, we redirect our thoughts to focus on something else. And that something else could be an eating issue of any sort; hence—eating disorders and aging meet.

Eating disorders are harder to diagnose in the older population because often they go undetected.

We think of eating disorders as mostly being the province of young teens and young adults, but this couldn't be further from the truth. In my practice I treat as many mature adults as I do teens. Why do we picture older adults free of such woes? Because we don't think of eating disorders and the older population in one breath. We imagine eating fixations as something that's outgrown as people march toward maturity.

Aging gets a bum rap. The elderly are thought of as frumpy, heavy, and not well groomed. So to counter this image others may have of them, many older people jump on the diet bandwagon, searching for youth in a harmful way through drastic measures.

These radical means of dealing with food could include extreme types of diets that might rebound in bouts of binge eating as a pacifier; or maybe an unaddressed, undiagnosed food addiction is lurking in the background. This doesn't need to be the case. Better ways of greeting our healthy older selves exist that result in no harm. And important to recall is that older adults have become a rapidly growing portion of the world's population.

Nutrition is a central determinant of physical and mental health, and plays a primary role in successful aging, according to Bulut, Khoury, et al. in the *Journal of Nutrition and Healthy Aging.* Food, to be discussed in Chapter 13, is key to the aging process.

The article by Bulut and others recognizes a decline in weight and energy intake with aging, coined as "anorexia of aging" as the most common eating disturbance in the elderly. Anorexia of aging is defined as the loss of appetite and/or decreased food intake in late life, a notable example of geriatric syndromes. Though this is a common occurrence, this type of progression with age isn't what I'm referring to. I'm looking at older individuals controlling their eating to mask the fear of aging

Though food intake undergoes substantial changes over the course of a life, here I'm talking about controlling eating as a means of addressing aging itself. Let's also note that poor nutritional status makes older adults more vulnerable to internal and/or external stressors, which can severely affect overall health and quality of life. Good nutrition, sufficient in terms of calories and vitamins, minerals, and such is essential because this gives individuals the opportunity to live healthier and longer lives.

Please note in this discussion I'm not referring to the frail elderly who are declining physically and mentally with no appetite, leading to increased malnutrition. And I'm not talking about a socioeconomic status in which food is scarce due to lack of income, or even the case of the elderly person isolated from friends and family dipping into depression. I'm talking about persons who manipulate their weight to feel and look younger. I'm talking about eating disorders that are overlooked in the older population.

A Quest for Thin and Young

I recall a beautiful woman, Antoinette, well into her fifties, a very chic, well-dressed, handsome woman, who summered at her vacation home on Martha's Vineyard, an island located south of Cape Cod in Massachusetts—an area known as being an affluent summer colony.

Antoinette was lovely in every sense, inside and out. But she had a big secret: She hated her body and feared aging and becoming fat. She came to me for therapy because she was obsessed with staying thin and young *at any cost.* She had childhood diabetes (Type I) that controlled her, day in and day out. She felt she had no escape until she learned to manipulate her insulin (diabulimia) and became quite thin, which took her mind onto a new fixation.

By manipulating her insulin, her blood glucose levels became elevated, and if they stayed that way, Antoinette would lose weight. At first she thought she'd made an amazing discovery, but she soon learned that doing this could evoke devastating and permanent effects on her body.

Antoinette was terrified, and made a frantic call for help. The early consequences she suffered from this behavior were dehydration, frequent urination, insatiable thirst, increased appetite, high blood-glucose levels, fatigue, and decreased concentration, along with electrolyte imbalance.

In addition to all this, Antoinette experienced insatiable hunger due to the manipulation, but the prize worth the discomfort, she thought at the time, was the weight loss. At first, she ignored the warnings that she was at risk of developing micro-vascular and macro-vascular complications, such as heart disease, stroke, neuropathy, retinopathy and nephropathy. What really got her attention, though, was the fact that she was at risk of early death if she continued this behavior. Of course, she did become very sick to the point she nearly lost a few of her toes. And to be honest, the thought of a disfigured body was what really woke her up.

This episode began for Antoinette as a *want to be thin*, but like many of us as we age, she began to fear not only her body not looking thin and toned, but now the fact that as she aged, she would look old. *And this is where the road of eating disorders and aging meet.*

Eating disorders are rough; I speak from experience. I wish I could have changed my thoughts back when my problems all began, but I didn't know I could, and I certainly didn't know how — and I definitely didn't know I could be happy. And as for Antoinette, she too had the same wonder, could she ever be happy in the body she had and not worry about weight and aging? And the answer was a resounding yes, she learned. I learned, and you can learn too, to embrace where you are in the here and now.

But though this change in attitude and approach aren't entirely easy, that someone can make up their mind to be happy and begin the process of igniting the happy spark is possible and feasible.

Louise L. Hay (may she rest in peace) wrote in *You Can Heal Your Life*, "What we think about ourselves becomes the truth for us." These words are key to turning your life around. If you "think" you're fat, or you're a loser, or any negative dialogue for that matter, you're setting up the possibility of becoming that person.

Louise played a huge role in my life as I battled with negative inner chatter, trying to come to terms with my eating disorder. I began reading her works as far back as 1976 *(Heal Your Body),* at a time when exploring the connection between the mind and body—let alone the spiritual component of that equation—wasn't popular. But even then, she was known as a motivational author who penned self-help advice. She was the guru of positive affirmations and self-healing.

Reading Louise Hay's works encouraged me to create joy in my life by recognizing the power of my thoughts as they related to my body and food challenges, and later, the aging process. In time, I began to grasp that I had control over the stories I created in my mind and I could use positive words to build positive stories.

Louise was known to frequently say, "All is well!"

Learning to work through mind mantras and change negative thoughts to positive ones kick starts the progression to releasing obsessions with negative inner diet chatter and begins your healing from the inside out.

Eating Disorders

Thus, as we navigate through releasing the obsession with aging, addressing the different eating disorders is both necessary and appropriate. Though many types of eating disorders exist, and often one blends with another — or one ends while another appears — I'm going to look at the four most common types of eating disorders defined in the *Diagnostic and Statistical Manual of Mental Disorders, Fifth Edition* (*DSM-5*).

Though I described diabulimia above, it is not an official eating disorder diagnosis or a medically recognized term, but it is used to describe an eating disorder suffered by someone with Type 1 diabetes, like Antoinette, who manipulated insulin to lose weight. It would fall under the category of bulimia through insulin manipulation.

The four most common eating disorders are: anorexia, binge eating, bulimia, and lastly other eating disorders characterized by some variants of the first three.

Briefly, anorexia nervosa can often be recognized in a person of low body weight that is unhealthy for their body type, height, or activity level. The anorexic restricts food, with achieving thinness as the main goal. This person harbors an intense fear of becoming fat. The inner chatter concerns the fear of "getting fat" and the person believes they are viewed as fat. This population is hyper-focused on calorie intake, body shape, and weight.

Bulimia nervosa, a second eating disorder, is noted as occurring in an individual eating large amounts of food, often in hiding (secret), and then purging through vomiting, laxatives, or extreme exercise. This type of eating-disordered person more often than not will binge and purge cyclically. They eat compulsively, binge eating well past the point of comfort.

The bulimic group typically practices a cycle of bingeing followed by fasting. They diet constantly while obsessing over their body weight and how they look. Those with this disorder can be of normal weight or overweight. They are not underweight, which is one of the differences between anorexia and bulimia.

The third eating disorder is binge eating disorder, oftentimes referred to as compulsive overeating — eating well beyond the point of fullness. This group of people may be overweight or obese and definitely feel out of control during a binge. Not uncommonly the binge eater will experience depression, anxiety, and feelings of isolation.

The fourth type of eating disorder is a "catch all" for all other eating disorders (and is called "other eating disorders"), their excess practices including extreme exercise and restrictive diets used solely to lose weight, such as veganism, a raw food diet, and/or only liquid diets. Other eating disorders also include late night binge eating, the use of diet pills, or any stimulant addiction with the purpose of speeding up metabolism in order to lose weight.

Food addiction, which falls in the "catch all" category, is named as "compulsive eating" rather than "food addiction." I call it what it is: food addiction. Food addiction constitutes an uncontrollable urge for excess food, particularly refined carbohydrates such as sugar and flour substances, which are quick to metabolize.

Food addiction, and/or a compulsion to eat, or any mixture of the eating disorders, often goes hand in hand with aging. How, you might ask? Well, food addicts and eating-disordered persons obsess about food, body, and looks. Aging addicts obsess about aging, and often they are the very same persons who began with eating issues.

The disease of food addiction—for food addiction truly constitutes a disease—is biochemical in nature because the body of the food addict reacts differently to certain foods than the bodies of other people. Food addicts obsess about their body size and what might happen if they are out of control with their food. And with that, often comes the fear of aging—hand in hand they go.

A common link behind food addictions is sensitivity to sugars and certain carbohydrates. More specifically, the reaction of deep craving begins with just one chocolate bar, a slice of cake, a bowl of pasta, or similar carbohydrates: *all normal foods for most individuals.*

After I struggled with my food addiction for well over thirty years, I found if I let go of my trigger foods, the monster within quieted. I began my personal journey by adopting a manner of eating in order to become "sober" and avoid relapse. I learned quickly that if I plugged into the universal life force and omitted processed foods, the demon was tamed, and I was relieved of the disease—yet I remained keenly aware that the consumption of sugar would open the mouth to the devil and ignite the addictive phase.

Compulsion is defined as a strong, usually irresistible, impulse to perform an act, especially one that is irrational or contrary to a person's ordinary state—and that leads one to become a sort of Dr. Jekyll and Mr. Hyde, living a double life. When the food addict eats the *strange potion*, otherwise known as simple carbohydrates, the person is transformed into a devilish creature who moves from being rational and "normal" to behaving as a raging, obnoxious fool—a tainted soul. Food addiction involves engaging—despite adverse consequences—in a continuous and compulsive use of food in an endless and incessant pursuit of a mood change.

Compulsion is always present in the disease of addiction, whether the addiction is to cocaine, vodka, or chocolate bars—or seeking to remain young.

For sugar-sensitive people, specific foods can be as enslaving as cocaine, alcohol, or any of the other substances that are addictive to some. Scientists such as Haddock and Dill (2000) have concluded certain food can be considered psychoactive, supporting the validity of the food addiction model. Moreover, the food addiction model is widely accepted by a portion of the general public—because it works when other understandings fail.

Addiction is the persistent and repetitive enactment of a behavioral pattern the person recurrently fails to resist and that consequently leads to significant physical, psychological, social, legal, or other major life problems. Loss of control over eating and obesity initiates changes in the brain similar to those produced by drugs of abuse.

Take this same thought and look at the compulsion or addictive tendency of the age-defiant person, who fears the aging process and is obsessed with stopping and controlling the inevitable progression to looking older. The anti-aging addiction also sparks the persistent and repetitive enactment of a behavioral pattern the person time and time again fails to resist and that consequently leads to significant physical, psychological, social, legal, or other major life problems. Though anti-aging behavior is not spurred by a chemical imbalance, as we see in an addict ingesting certain foods, anti-aging behaviors cause a "lighting up" in the brain at the thought of looking young if we do this or that...

Binge eaters and drug abusers commonly report an undeniable yearning to consume the substance *no matter what* the cost. The feeling is the same for those possessed by the idea of fighting aging—no matter what the cost. Binge eating is a prominent feature of many eating disorders and shares many diagnostics with substance abuse. Binge eaters, similar to excessive drinkers, prefer privacy and isolation and an element of secrecy prior to and during a binge.

Of course age-obsessed persons are not isolating IF they find the solution or correction for all the world to see. At that point, they'll leave the safety and privacy of their cocoons and enter into a social atmosphere for the oohs and ahs...the same recognition the newly thin body craves after a restriction of some sort.

Considerable research evidence supports a genetic component to the development of eating disorders. As is seen in many other types of disturbances of normal functioning, eating disorders cluster in families. Twin studies consistently furnish evidence that eating disorders may be inherited. Recent research suggests that biological relatives of those with eating disorders run a five- to 12-fold times the normal risk of also developing an eating disorder.

A Recap

Eating disorders affect people of *all* ages, genders, and races. Seniors are often at risk of disordered eating patterns due to the emotional and physical changes they face as they age. Though eating disorders are dangerous as a whole, this can be even more true with elders who may have compromised health to begin with. Added to other health problems, disordered eating can be dangerous, as eating disorders directly alter health.

Not uncommonly, anorexia nervosa can be seen when seniors rigidly restrict their food intake. This extreme control of eating in older persons often is triggered by depression, loneliness, or fears of aging, rather than the usual compulsive desire to be thin.

Bulimia, as noted earlier, most often involves purging after meals by either vomiting or abusing laxatives. These practices aren't always easy to spot because bulimia doesn't normally result in drastic weight loss or changes in eating patterns, alerting others—especially with the older population. As with any bulimic behavior (even one like Antoinette's diabulimia) bulimia is dangerous for everyone, but especially for seniors because the repeated purging may lead to dehydration, gastritis, and heart problems.

Along with anorexia and bulimia (and food addiction) is binge eating, which is characterized by periods when seniors quickly and uncontrollably eat overwhelmingly large amounts of food. Binge eating disorder often occurs alongside anorexia or bulimia, but the older population with this issue tends to gain an unhealthy amount of weight due to a sedentary lifestyle.

Another eating disorder that may go undetected with the older population is orthorexia, characterized by an overwhelming preoccupation with health that leads to severely restricting their diet to only foods they consider healthy. On the surface, eating only healthful foods looks like a great plan, but with orthorexia a restriction can become quite serious because often the orthorexic may gradually cut out almost all food groups until they're down to a small category of "safe foods" such as raw vegetables. In time, such disordered and obsessive eating patterns can lead to unhealthy weight loss or behavioral issues.

Orthorexia is closely linked to obsessive-compulsive disorders and is not too far from food addiction, all of which usually require psychotherapy to combat. And the aging population may hook into this type of eating disorder as an attempt to manipulate the aging process with rules regarding good and bad foods. Now, this is not to be confused with food addicts who refrain from sugar, flour, and wheat to reign in the addictive eating in the same way an alcoholic would stop drinking to stop the compulsion for more alcohol.

So, I think I've made evident that eating disorders are not just for the teenager and young adult, but they also plague the mature adult, still looking for thin, young, and even some kind of rejuvenation. Though older populations may undertake a reduced degree of exercise and fewer binge episodes, bulimia nervosa, nonetheless, presents across all age groups without regard to demographics (race, gender, or marital status) in terms of fasting, self-induced vomiting, and laxative use.

And now that we've looked at eating disorders and aging, diving into food, mood, and wrinkles in Chapter 13 makes perfect sense.

Personal Inventory Questions

1. Have you ever been beckoned to come to the edge but something inside warned you not to, for fear of falling or some type of change you thought you couldn't handle… and then you dipped your toe in, and it wasn't so bad after all? Go back into your earliest memory and recall what that experience was like. Was it as frightening, or as earth shattering as you feared?

2. In my case, and that of most of my patient load, and possibly for you, the reader, fear of aging started with the fear of not being in control as life began to change — way back when we were tiny, little people. Perhaps we thought we could at least control our bodies when we couldn't control life challenges. Is this true for you?

3. Eating disorders are harder to detect in the older population because they are an unexpected type of problem. We think of eating disorders only in the young teen and young adult, but this couldn't be further from the truth. What are your experiences with aging and eating disorders?

4. Aging gets a bum rap, that with it we become frumpy, heavy, and not well groomed. So to counter this, many jump on the diet bandwagon, searching for youth in a harmful way through drastic measures.

5. By manipulation of insulin, the blood glucose levels can become elevated, and if they stay there, the diabetic can lose weight. At first Antoinette

thought she made an amazing discovery, but she soon learned devastating and permanent bodily effects could result. Have you done something drastic to manipulate your weight? If so, what was the outcome, and what did you learn from it?

6. The four most common eating disorders are: anorexia, binge eating, bulimia — and lastly — "other" eating disorders, characterized by some variants of the first three. Did you ever have an eating disorder? If so, how did it play out for you and did you outgrow it?

7. Food addiction is defined as an uncontrollable urge for excess food, particularly refined carbohydrates such as sugar and flour substances, which are quick to metabolize. Have you ever known yourself to have food sensitivities? Do certain foods cause you to binge eat?

8. Binge eaters and drug abusers commonly report an undeniable yearning to consume the substance *no matter what* the cost. Similarly, those obsessed with fighting aging will do so no matter the cost. What price will you pay for youth? What price will you pay for a thin quest?

9. Considerable research evidence supports a genetic component to the development of eating disorders. As is seen in many other types of disturbances of normal functioning, eating disorders cluster in families. If you look at your genetics, do you see eating disorders in family members? Look up, down, and

sideways…grandparents, uncles, cousins, children…

10. Another eating disorder that may go undetected with the older population is orthorexia, an overwhelming preoccupation with health and severely restricting their diet to foods they consider healthy. Are you on a "healthy" food kick, which limits your variety of foods? What foods are "okay" and which are not?

Chapter 13

Food, Mood, and Wrinkles

People are like stained glass windows.
They sparkle and shine when the sun is out,
but when the darkness sets in,
their true beauty is revealed
only if there is a light from within.
~Elisabeth Kubler-Ross

When darkness sets in, and we are no longer in our youth, what beauty is revealed? Is it a beauty that's coming from within? Seasons come and seasons go — and within each, comes learning, a growing. When we peel away the outer layers, we have only what's within. We no longer ride on the coattails of outer beauty, but now look deeply into our souls.

Beauty has always been from within, but when the sun is shining and all the wonder of life's promises is ahead of us, we might miss such wisdom. Do we need life's hard knocks to learn this? Perhaps yes, but maybe no. We can find the torch of love within if we open our hearts and look beyond outer beauty. This is not always an easy or comfortable task. And then, when our mood is added to the mix, the issue of beauty can be more complicated.

And to take the question a step beyond outer and inner beauty, the food we eat plays a role in both. For years, I've studied the part food and mood contribute in regard to eating disorders, but now I'm looking through another lens as I age and those I work with are aging, too. Ethnicity, wealth, and education don't count much when the matter comes to mood and food; the chemical connection with the sustenance that fuels us is what will make us, or break us.

Though we touched on food in Chapter 7, Genetics vs. Lifestyle, and a discussion of diet is threaded throughout this book, I want to take a closer look at how food affects both our mood and our appearance. This chapter examines food and the chemicals known as neurotransmitters in our brain.

Some foods cause a high while others cause a low in moods. Some foods can work like drugs affecting our mood, which can lead to stress, which can add to the aging process, as hinted at in earlier chapters.

We also explored eating disorders and how they work alongside the aging process, but now we're looking at food addiction and/or food sensitivity. In addition, we're examining processed versus unprocessed foods and how they work on our mood and show on us physically—whether we radiate health, or not—hence: food, mood, and wrinkles.

Food definitely plays a key role in our moods *and* in our physical appearance. For some, whether in their youth or older age, particular foods can be as addictive as cocaine. And for others, the question isn't about the addictive foods, but rather the choice of foods. In addition, as we age, medications can take a role in the food and mood issue.

The Meds Made Me Do It

One of my sisters had an allergic reaction to a plant similar to poison ivy,

a woody shrub or small tree, known as poison sumac. When exposed, she broke out in a rash over her entire body, to the point that she needed medical assistance. She was put on prednisone, along with calamine lotion, and became agitated and unable to sleep though she was normally a very good sleeper. She also became ravenous, and she noticed a shift in her mood.

While the focus here is on aging and the role of food from a mood perspective, at the same time, as we age, we can have a change in diet, medical issues, or medications, all of which may wreak havoc on our moods.

My father always ate the Mediterranean diet with lots of fresh fruits, vegetables, a wide source of protein, nuts, olive oil on anything he could drizzle it over, along with drinking wine. His skin was smooth and radiant until the latter part of his life.

As my father entered his mid-eighties, he was put on Coumadin, a common name for warfarin, an anticoagulant (blood thinner), known to reduce the formation of blood clots to reduce the risk of stroke, heart attack, or other serious conditions. This medication works by decreasing the effectiveness of vitamin K. In other words it works by inhibiting the action of vitamin K in the liver.

Normally, vitamin K helps your blood clot so wounds don't bleed too much, but Coumadin (warfarin) works against vitamin K, making your blood clot more slowly. In other words, Coumadin and vitamin K work against each other. Because of this, keeping a balance is important—not suddenly eating a lot more or a lot less vitamin K-rich foods than normal for that person.

So for my father to eat a balanced source of vitamin K in his diet–green leafy vegetables such as spinach, kale, broccoli and parsley—was essential. High levels of Coumadin, especially with a low vitamin K intake, have the potential to cause severe bleeding from a wound, nosebleed, or various types of internal bleeding. My father began to cough up blood from time to time, and was known to have nosebleeds.

To make matters more complicated, my father had terrible pains in his stomach when he ate strawberries or foods with seeds. He had a condition that began when small bulging pouches (diverticula) developed in his digestive tract. But in time, more and more of the pouches became inflamed, turning his condition into diverticulitis.

Our diets are connected to our moods and mental acuity; if the diet changes drastically, it affects not only our mindset, but our physical appearance, too. My father had beautiful skin all the way to the end of his life (at ninety-one), not a wrinkle to be found because he ate well in his earlier years. However, in his later years, his gait slowed, his balance become wobbly, and his diet was atrocious—by choice, not recommendation—and his thoughts became cloudy and sometimes confused.

My father's healthy Mediterranean diet went out the window as he sought crackers, gelatin-type foods, doughnuts, and cookies for nutrition. He turned away from foods rich in vitamin K. He wasn't advised to eat poorly, but one medication required one type of diet, while the complications that come with diverticulitis required another—at least back then. At that time the doctors advised that he avoid nuts, seeds, zucchini, cucumbers, strawberries, and raspberries along with red meats, all foods he loved.

Are We What We Eat?
Are we what we eat? Seemingly so. I recall a crazy diet I was on many moons ago; it consisted of loads of carrots. In time, I began to look a bit orange and felt agitated. During another period, I ate pure junk on a bender for days on end. Boils, causing excruciating pain, popped up on my body.

At another stage of my life, I was on a crazy Ritz cracker and cream cheese diet (don't try this!!) drinking only hot tea — and soon, my complexion was that of a soggy Ritz. Or how about the time I was on diet pills and my face was full of pimples, and I was higher than a kite.

Could food dictate our mood — our wrinkles? If I ate cardboard for breakfast, lunch, and dinner, would that show in the shade of my complexion, increasing lines and signs of aging, just as the Ritz did? And what about my father eating Mediterranean most of his life and having amazing skin along with a great attention span and even-tempered moods — with the exception of the normal Italian flare-up from time to time.

If we are what we eat, then perhaps the foods rich in nutrients play a huge part in contributing to healthier skin and happier self. On a diet of fewer natural foods, my father soon became confused, talked less and less, and slept more and more. For sure, he was getting up in years, but I'm convinced the food played a huge role in his rapid decline.

Are we like stained glass windows? Do we sparkle and shine when the sun is out? And when darkness sets in, is our true beauty revealed — if there is a light within? So often the metaphor of a light within to show beauty from the inside to the outside is touted. We live between two worlds, our inside world and the world we show the outside, and often they're not one and the same. But when they are, the effect is powerful and magical.

In Chapter 10, we discussed eating disorders and aging, and how the two roads meet. Now we turn our attention to foods, mood, and aging combined. The outcome can be positive as we saw in Chapter 7, when Aiden turned to healthy, real foods.

No doubt the food we eat is paramount in our healthy aging as it plays out in our mood and our exterior presentation. Food can act as a mood stabilizer, and in some cases, for those addicted to certain foods; it can perform as a drug.

Food, a Mood Stabilizer

That unhealthy eating patterns can cause mood swings at any age is no secret. Why? Well, blood sugar fluctuations and nutritional imbalances are often to blame. We need a continuous steady source of *real* fuel from the foods we eat in order for our minds and bodies to function well. And often people have food sensitivities that cause erratic and addictive behavior.

During my research, interviews, and work with eating disordered patients prior to writing my first book, *Release Your Obsession with Food: Heal from the Inside Out,* I explored the experience of food addiction; learning addiction to food was not so different from substance or alcohol addictions. I found that food, for some, was similar, if not identical, to other addictions and was described in similar ways. Words such as "sober," "intoxicated," and "substance" were brought up when those with food addiction would describe how some foods made them feel. The section below is from *Release Your Obsession with Food.*

I conducted my interviews based on questions as to how the food sensitive person felt, and this is what I learned from people collectively. Certain foods were described by those interviewed as *drugs*, even by those who were in recovery from drug addiction. On many days, "We were so hung over from a binge, we couldn't perform simple tasks such as answer the phone, return calls, make appointments, or show up for engagements—and all the while we hid our addictions. Isolation protected us."

All those I spoke to reacted to certain foods as if they were drugs, creating mood alterations powerful enough to hold each in a pattern of binge eating despite their best efforts to try and break the behavior. "These foods for us *are* drugs; through chemical reactions, they eventually cause a production of brain chemicals that have a drug-like effect on the body."

These brain chemicals are known as neurotransmitters. A neurotransmitter is a chemical substance that carries impulses from one nerve cell to another. They act as messages within the brain, which help control the body.

I learned when we (including me) made a beeline for crackers, pasta, bread, pretzels, or any other simple carbohydrate while experiencing anxiety, tension, or irritable moods, we were most likely looking for serotonin—a nerve chemical (neurotransmitter) that turns on when these foods are metabolized. We were self-medicating, and temporarily, we would feel calm.

Our bodies naturally make serotonin but some of us don't produce enough. Antidepressant medications such as Celexa, Cymbalta, Prozac, and Paxil, to name a few, are used to increase the serotonin. Serotonin plays a huge role in mood and appetite.

Cravings for starches and sweets can turn on and off, depending on the level of serotonin, which regulates mood, sleep cycles, memory, and pain tolerance. Relatively high levels of serotonin have a calming effect that lead to a clearer mind and stable mood. Low levels of serotonin sink the mood, and clarity is lost—hence, a binge to knock us out of our pain and agitation.

Dopamine and norepinephrine are other neurotransmitters that also play key roles in regard to food and mood. For instance, low levels of these neurotransmitters, like low levels of serotonin, are associated with an increase in depression. Increasing dopamine and norepinephrine improves mood, alertness, mental clarity, and the ability to cope with stress. Foods higher in protein will raise the dopamine and norepinephrine levels.

Though all these hormones may have similar effects, helping with mental clarity, reducing depression and anxiety, and stabilizing mood, excessive serotonin can result in sleep disturbances, insomnia, irritability, and mental confusion. For the food addict, too much in the way of simple carbohydrates will drastically increase the level of serotonin, leading to these negative effects. Eating adequate amounts of protein is critical for the food addict then to bring down the high serotonin and normalize moods.

Not uncommon is for food addicts to fill up on pancakes laced with syrup to increase their serotonin levels and then go for a sizzling steak to pull down the serotonin, hence vacillating between highs and lows — *uppers and downers.*

Chocolate, which contains phenyl ethylamine (PEA), a substance that stimulates the release of dopamine, also helps regulate the mood and explains chocolate cravings. Chocolate, in fact, often serves as an anodyne — a self-medication — to relieve distress or pain that we can't even put our finger on. We ignore our dark emotions and feed ourselves instead, as a balm, which eventually leads to furthering our addictions. The cravings and increased consumption may well be a last-ditch effort to regulate moods.

The revelation in regard to food sensitivity is that food addiction isn't necessarily a psychological habit or stemming from past traumatic experiences — it's a chemical reaction. As noted above, many mood alterations result from imbalances in the neurotransmitters and other hormones that regulate behavior.

One doesn't have to be a food addict to feel the up and down with moods and food. Mood swings with food could be food sensitivity or a lack of whole foods. Age knows no bias to these mood fluctuations.

Chemical levels of emotion-altering agents such as serotonin, dopamine, and endorphins can be dramatically affected by a single meal or a change in dietary habits. Cravings for foods such as sweets, starches, caffeine, and chocolate (to name a few) originate in fundamental biological drives to improve our moods.

Keep It Real

Threaded throughout the chapters in this book, I point to the importance of eating real, natural, whole foods as essential to your overall wellbeing. The time has arrived for all of us to take charge of the foods we eat. The Standard American Diet is known as SAD, which true to the acronym is truly disheartening because SAD is mostly made up of processed foods that include artificial color, additives, flavorings, and chemically altered fats and sweeteners.

Our brains cannot detect these foods as real, giving our bodies the wrong signals instead of the nutrients we need to feed the trillion cells the human body is composed of. Cells are the basic building blocks of all living things. They provide structure for the body, take in nutrients from food, convert nutrients into energy, and carry out specialized functions. If we are not inputting real food, the brain is confused and doesn't know where to allocate this fake food.

The reason food is so vital to getting these nutrients to our cells is that our bodies have evolved to "recognize" the nutrients they can extract from whole foods. When my father's foods went from real to fake, the change was drastic and the result showed almost instantly. Knowing real from not real foods is simple. Does it come off a tree, out of the ground, fly in the air, roam on the land, or swim in the sea? Then, it's real. Does it come in packages, cans, or wrappers, then it might not be so real. Will your food rot? Or will it last for months on end — it's probably not real if it lasts.

Little efforts we put forth can make all the difference in how we age even when we think the endeavors are so small they can't possibly slow down the aging process or improve how we look. Think again. Here's a basket of opportunity for us when we put forth the effort. You'll see in Chapter 14 as we *Turn the Corner* and explore how little efforts go a long way.

Personal Inventory Questions
1. "People are like stained glass windows. They sparkle and shine when the sun is out, but when darkness sets in, their true beauty is revealed only if there is a light from within." (Elisabeth Kubler-Ross). Do you feel a light from within? How do you tap into your inner beauty?
2. Are we what we eat? I recall a crazy diet I was on many moons ago that consisted of loads of carrots. In time I began to look a bit orange and felt agitated. Can you recall a crazy way you ate in the past? How did it impact your mood — your aging?

3. Yes, food definitely plays a key role in our moods and in our physical appearance. For some, foods can be as addictive as cocaine, whether in their youth or older age. Do you have a food addiction or sensitivity to food? If so, how does it affect you?

4. Maybe for you the question is not the addictive nature of the foods, but rather the choice of foods. What foods do you tend to head for? We all have our go-to foods, so what are yours?

5. As we age, medications and diet can play a role in the food and mood cycle. Are you on medication? Does it affect your food choices or your mood?

6. Our diet is connected to our mood, and if the diet changes drastically, the change can affect not only our mindset, but our physical appearance too. I mentioned the mental and physical changes that took place with my father when he changed his diet. Have you noticed a change caused by your food? Explore the changes.

7. I conducted interviews based on questions as to how the food sensitive person felt. Certain foods were described by those interviewed as drugs, even by those who were in recovery from drug addiction. What resonated with you in considering the power of neurotransmitters—the chemicals in our brain?

8. Relatively high levels of serotonin have a calming effect that lead to a clearer mind and stable mood. Low levels of serotonin sink the mood and clarity is lost—hence, a binge may follow to knock us out

of our pain and agitation. Which foods do you lean toward?

9. Have you noticed certain foods make you happy, while others make you sad, and still others make you feel irritable? Make a list of the foods that you eat and associate what moods are triggered by each.

10. Aging is inevitable, but clearly our food plays a huge role. Which food do you eat that leave you looking and feeling radiant?

Part III

Turn the Corner

Chapter 14

Little Things Do Count

*Whether you think you can or think you can't,
you're right.*
~Henry Ford

Whether you think you can or think you can't, you're right.
If you believe you can't do something, whatever that
something is, you've set yourself up for failure. And
whatever you think you can do opens the door for
great possibilities. The more you do, the more you can
do—and with that in mind, little things add up to big
change when you start with small steps. From this
point, you're *turning the corner* to final steps to
releasing your obsession with aging.

With a little effort, the aging process can go
smooth as silk, most often depending on you and

what you do, sans an illness or accident. Think of this chapter as a basket of tricks that will lead to youthful appearance and behavior — naturally. The basket contains Basic Grooming 101 tips that will make you feel better, look better, and present whole and healthy.

Where to begin in such a discussion is ammunition for an entire book in and of itself. I'm not sure one chapter can do the topic justice, but it's definitely a spark to ignite a big change for you. Believing little efforts really don't count or add up to much is easy, but the reality can't be further from the truth.

Take writing for example. Many of my friends are writers, and most have a daily writing schedule they plan to implement. But often the time comes and goes, and no writing work is accomplished, creating a bundle of guilt and self-doubt.

In my writing groups, writers often present the question, "How many words do you write a day?" I hear answers such as, "I plan 2,000 words a day, but somehow I'm sidetracked, or I can't think of what to write — can't find my muse."

I've never been one to write for hours on end every day, but rather I put forth a 500-words-a-day schedule. That's it. I only expect to write 500 words, and more often than not, that 500 turns into thousands.

Why is that so? Well, I believe that's the case because I don't feel any pressure. Knocking out 500 words and ending there is easy for me. And then that

500 often starts the juices flowing, and before I know it, I've written a great deal, leading to another completed book.

And so, this is what I mean by little things do count. If we take steps toward basic daily improvements, those actions will become our norm, leading us to a ritual of practices we'll soon carry out automatically — and NOT obsessively.

So where do we begin with the basket of tricks in an effort to slow down the aging process, or to present ourselves as being more youthful? I say grooming is a great place to start. Basic grooming consists of: bathing, brushing teeth, combing or brushing hair, and much more. Now you may be rolling your eyes, thinking everyone bathes and brushes their teeth and that this is a silly start to a chapter.

Grooming 101

Grooming 101 is a basket of suggestions that might surprise you and lead you to a more youthful you. We'll look at how bathing, brushing teeth, dressing appropriately, and so on, to name a few, bring out your sexy and spirituality.

Now you may be the sort who's pristine and well-put-together. We all know the type: You throw on a scarf, a little lipstick, diamond studs, and you are so ready to go— but some of us just aren't natural fashionistas with a grooming touch.

Good hygiene starts with making sure your ears are clean — and for you gentlemen, the hair is removed—and from your nose too. Gigi was a fun, loving, laugh-easy type, who was ready to date. She was a stunning beauty with crisp white hair, piercing blue eyes, and a smile that would blow any guy away. Gigi wanted to find Mr. Right during her eighty-first year on this earth.

Our girl looked on every dating site and found one frog after another, but no prince. One fellow she really liked, but he didn't smell of cologne; he believed the natural scent was best. Gigi stomped into my office, really agitated. "This guy is perfect in every way, but he has hair in his nose and ears, and smells like wet bark." Done, she was done.

I also recall Marla, a nurse practitioner who met Roger; a dashing cardiologist with dimples the size of grapes and perfect, all-white teeth to go with them. He was everything she was looking for—until he ate. On their first date, she excused that he licked his fingers after each bite of his succulent barbeque chicken wings, but when he made the same move after eating a salad, she was finished. Speaking to me in a loud tone, she asked, "What kind of momma raises her boy to lick his fingers while eating?"

I'm not sure the finger-licking was his momma's fault but for sure this was a habit Marla wasn't willing to accept.

And then John met Sally, a match made in heaven. She cooked and wore high heels, while her nails were flawlessly shaped and her fingernail polish was never chipped. She was perfect. She laughed at all of John's silly jokes and shared his same passion for gardening and taking long walks along the beach. Sally was every man's dream, but she often skipped brushing her teeth and wasn't interested in flossing or whitening them. When she bent forward to kiss John, he was subjected to a whiff of sour milk left out for days. This was a deal breaker for John.

Peter met Betty, who was as cute as a button. She loved to dance and go out to dinner with his friends, and she fit right in. She contributed to deep conversations and left the group smiling, as she was warm and funny with smarts to match. So, what could be wrong with Betty, as she's sounding so perfect? She was — *almost* — but Betty didn't believe in shaving. Her legs were as hairy as Peter's dog Bo, and under her arms was a patch, resembling a man's pits, not to mention the moustache she had going above her lips. These details weren't working for Peter, and Betty wasn't willing to change and join the majority of American women who remove hairy parts.

Now if you personally choose not to brush your teeth or make your pearly whites white, or you want hair to grow freely in all parts, by all means have at it, but keep in mind your significant other's wish may not be down with that. And that's okay, because someone's taste may well coincide with yours; the search may just take a longer while. That said, if you want to feel fresh and youthful, and present that too, then you might want to tap into Basic Grooming 101. Just say'n.

A Little Bath Anyone?

You might be surprised to learn some of us don't bathe regularly, and as we age, maybe that occurs even less often. Why? Possibly the older person is afraid of falling, or standing in the shower is difficult, or they might not have the energy. A cultural factor may also be involved, or someone might not bathe due to issues related to poverty or lack of access to water in abundance. When the matter is survival, a roof over our heads, food, and drinking water take precedence over general hygiene.

But for most here in the U.S. of A, plenty of water is available for basic hygiene. Overall, this section is meant for those who just don't bathe *because they just don't bathe,* not due to economics or a cultural belief system. And for the record, most people DO bathe, but not all. I can think of many — *many* older persons who don't bathe daily for one reason or another — and that's fine. But not bathing isn't fine when it affects your overall health, mentally, physically or emotionally.

Simply put, washing and bathing are the most important ways to maintain good health and protect us from infections, illnesses, and so on. Keeping the body surface clean prevents dirt from being trapped in scabs, sores, or any open wound. In addition, basic hygiene — maintaining cleanliness — is also important for our emotional wellbeing, from a pride in our physical appearance to a sense of normal self-confidence.

Let's face it; the main purpose of washing is to remove dirt and odors. If we smell offensive, we aren't going to be invited or welcomed by others into their space—nor might we invite them into our own territory.

But regarding that same sense of things, some experts do say daily showering is not so necessary. Normal healthy skin maintains a layer of oil and a balance of "good" bacteria and other microorganisms, according to Robert H. Shmerling, M.D., senior faculty editor of *Harvard Health*, as he posts on the Harvard Health Blog. Washing and scrubbing removes these healthful bacteria, especially if the water is hot, he warns. Skin can become dry, irritated, or itchy. Not good.

His article goes on to say that approximately two-thirds of Americans shower daily, whereas in places such as China, about half of the population report bathing only twice a week. Who has this right? Showering seems to be more about habit and societal norms than health.

Okay so now what—do we bathe or not? Consider that if you smell, and it's offensive, maybe this is a no-brainer—take a bath. But if you shower in hot water and your skin becomes dry, the skin may crack, allowing infections and allergic reactions to surface.

Okay, so maybe wash the skin in warm, not hot, water and perhaps rinse up in between, if that's your preference. But you, the reader, might be like me, the writer, and think yuck, not showering doesn't seem right. And that's okay too. We can all agree if we're smelly and offensive, we might want to regroup and make some changes. How we achieve that change is up to us, individually.

Pursuing this consideration, the first person who comes to mind is a fellow I'll call Jeb, who I saw in my practice many years ago. He was thoughtful and kind, a real delight to work with—but—he would leave my office and the nastiest smell seemed to stay for hours on end.

I ran around spraying disinfectants, carpet powder, and even went so far as to purchase a continuous air freshener to spritz every few minutes (which sadly I had to remove because the spritz sound startled patients), and tried every other trick in the book to neutralize my room, to no avail. Jeb was considerate, smart, funny, and quite interesting to talk to, but he came in with a smell that stayed trapped in my room, *for days on end.* What to do?

Well, let's explore the reason I was seeing Jeb in the first place. Though many issues bubbled up, the one chief complaint for him in life was he wanted a close partner to share his life and dreams with, and he wasn't having much luck in that department. Okay...you can see where this is going. After my cautious, sensitive leading questions, he admitted one day he hadn't taken a shower in at least three months.

I wanted to shout out, "Aha, I knew it!!" But, of course I could not and would not do that because my work is to build confidence not tear it down. With gentle probing, he confessed he didn't think life was worth much for him, and that he didn't care. Jeb suffered from depression, anxiety, and posttraumatic stress disorder after serving in Vietnam in his teens. And with this information, I was finally able to assess and guide Jeb.

Mental illness can make its way into a personal life causing great havoc in so many parts of one's activities, even areas such as showering and brushing your teeth. And this was exactly what had happened to Jeb. Did I mention Jeb wasn't brushing? And did I mention Jeb's teeth were shifting and in risk of decaying?

Jeb was shutting down—or should I say he had shut down. Not that Jeb was lazy, or uneducated or suffering from poverty; no, that wasn't the cause of the problem at all. Jeb, along with a multitude of people, had a mental illness that was never addressed, until we began our work together.

Jeb was a prisoner in his own mind from unexamined and unresolved issues of long ago. As time marched on, with the compilation of life's' challenges, and not addressing the ghosts in the closet, he, in time, became a shell of a person, apathetic—really due to a suppression of passion, emotion, or any type of excitement. Jeb had taken on the appearance of an old man, hunched over, shuffling in and out of my office.

With some trepidation, I cautiously proceeded to discuss the importance of self-love and self-care, for Jeb himself, not for others, and that in time this would open doors to many positive experiences. We talked in depth about where his struggles were stemming from and began to unravel his traumas during his military service, which he'd never discussed with anybody, not ever. I gently probed and was able to discuss the possibility that we might talk further about this trauma he'd experienced. He was willing.

I'm happy to report the next week Jeb came in squeaky clean and fresh smelling. He walked taller, smiled freely, and said he felt much, much better. He also made an appointment with his dentist to discuss repairing his teeth. Today, Jeb has pearly whites and a life partner and works on basic grooming without any defensive resistance. He's happier and more confident than I'd ever known him to be. He looks youthful, wants to take adventurous trips, and lives a full life.

Yes, simple bathing can be key to overall health and wellbeing, and exploring the reasons for not wanting to work on self-hygiene can be the key to unlocking blockage of deeply hidden tragedies in life. Often we think, "I got this!" when in fact we don't; our old conflicts may be long buried, and not allowing us to live our best life.

What's A Bra Got to Do with It?

On this same note, a lovely, well-endowed redhead about to turn 60 years old, Molly, came to my office. She was a *hotty* in every sense of the word. She was tall, lean, with almond-shaped gold-flecked eyes, chiseled chin, turned-up button nose (the one I always dreamed of having), and she had a presence about her. She *really* was a head turner.

But when we first started working together, I noted that she didn't appear to be engaging in basic grooming. This is always a touchy subject to address, so I tiptoed around it, careful not to hurt her feelings. I soon learned money was not what kept her from seeking dental work, haircuts, or stylish clothes and good bras, as she had plenty. Her stumbling block was rather complacency. Now please don't think I'm the fashion police as you read this because I'm not. I'm *very* casual, but grooming...yes that's important.

As I gently queried, Molly admitted that she felt no need to bother with her grooming at her age because "Who'd want an old lady anyway?" She said this while laughing. She really had bought into the idea that over sixty meant old. Molly didn't suffer from depression or anxiety or poverty, so none of those were reasons for her to neglect her basic needs. She was of a solid healthy weight, so she didn't offer the excuse of having so much weight to lose that the battle was endless.

No, Molly was blessed with amazing genes, giving her a healthy body and tremendous looks. Did I mention she was a size double D in bra measurements, which got her more than a bit of attention? She was quite the looker, but didn't see it in herself. She just didn't think anybody would want a sixty-year-old woman. She only came to me because she wanted to quit smoking.

Yep, Molly was a smoker, and a heavy one at that. So, we had our work cut out for us. We started with brief psychotherapy that moved into hypnotherapy for the cessation of smoking. The reason she wanted to quit smoking was that she did have cancer in her family and feared it would get her if she kept pressing her luck. And besides, when she was a young girl she'd always promised she'd quit when she got old. So, now was the time and she was ready and determined.

Our work was quick in that after only three sessions, Molly quit smoking—just like that. But our success opened up a curiosity about what else she could accomplish since she had been able to let go of such a gripping, addictive, nasty habit (her words not mine). Ah, so with this opening, I snuck in basic grooming in a kindly way. We talked about building confidence physically, mentally, and spiritually, a trio that leads to amazing, miraculous results. Molly didn't believe we connect to any higher source, so we started there.

Warning, this is not a religious push by any means, but rather I want to discuss spirituality…and in the upcoming chapter we'll talk about, earth, God, spiritual connections and how these may or may not impact your life, but for now my focus is on the idea of reaching into that part of you that's connected to something, whatever that something is.

According to the online *Oxford English Dictionary*, spirituality is the quality of being concerned with the human spirit or soul, as opposed to material or physical things. Spirituality is a shift, so to speak, in priorities, that allows us to embrace the human essence in a more profound way.

Spirituality is a broad concept with loads of room for many perspectives, which is why I will cover it here loosely, as it's personal and defined differently by each individual. But for all, spirituality includes a sense of connection to something bigger than ourselves, and it typically involves a search for meaning in life, a topic we've talked about at length more than once in this book. Our own finding of the significance of each of our lives is, for me, a theme that spreads throughout the pages here even if only at a hint. A search for why we're in born bodies is a universal human pursuit that touches us all.

So we tapped into Molly's belief system, and she realized what she wanted to look into was not others' ideas of spirituality, but the one she might own for herself. She soon realized she had been taught that she wasn't to feel sexy or beautiful, as that was a sin; hence, she didn't wear good bras, causing her breasts to drop and nearly touch her belly button. We moved past that religious conditioning into how letting her natural beauty shine through with some attention to basic body needs would feel.

The first need we closed in on was for her to have a good bra that actually fit and lifted. The change once she was able to purchase such an item was short of miraculous. From there, we moved on to her having a fresh haircut to show off her natural curls. After those two great successes, Molly took off like wildfire, addressing her teeth, donning a pair of high heels, and finding a job as a personal assistant to a very well-to-do guy, a guy she actually eventually married.

How Are Your Pearly Whites?

Teeth play a huge role in the aging process for many reasons. For basics, taking care of your mouth, teeth, and gums is a worthy goal in and of itself. I learned this young, witnessing my mom who didn't take care of her teeth because she was afraid of the dentist. By the time she was in her fifties, she had dentures. I was determined to not go down that road.

But despite our very good intentions, life happens on life's terms, and I developed gum disease. How you might ask? In my case, I thought I inherited it. I also was broke during my twenties and thirties, leaving little money for dental care. Also, if you remember, I'm a food addict in recovery, and I spent a period of years eating loads of sugar-laden foods while not tending to my teeth, as I should have. Many eating disorder patients from bulimia to binge eating, and every type in between, neglect their teeth.

While I was fortunate enough to inherit straight, strong teeth with only two cavities in my life thus far, the gums didn't fare too well, to the point that I had gum surgery in one quadrant of my mouth. I was to have the remaining three quadrants, but miraculously they healed. How? I'm not sure if that was because I invested time in flossing, used a Waterpik, and did some serious brushing with a sonic electric brush, or if it's from the human growth hormone (HGH) gel I mentioned earlier. In any case, my gums are good today, not bleeding and not receding.

So again, taking diligent care of your mouth, teeth, and gums is worth its weight in gold, really. In addition, good oral and dental hygiene can prevent bad breath, tooth decay, and gum disease—and drum roll—can help you keep your teeth as you age. Regular brushing removes the plaque that causes tooth decay and stimulates your gums to help prevent gum disease.

Of course regular visits to the dentist is crucial in that it can lead to early disease detection. I generally go for a cleaning every three months without fail, even though my hygienist, Maria, said I could push it to four months. I'm not willing to take the chance. During the pandemic shutdown, however, I wasn't able to go in for my three-month visit, and to my joy, I had very little plaque after six months! Yes, regular, routine cleaning is wise and beneficial.

In addition, regular dental visits open the opportunity for your hygienist and dentist to catch issues early. For example they can discover through examination if you have:

✓ Heart problems
✓ Acid reflux
✓ Vitamin deficiencies
✓ Tooth grinding
✓ Osteoporosis
✓ Oral cancer

✓ Dementia
✓ Mental health issues
✓ Eating disorders
✓ Diabetes

Worse, ignoring our oral hygiene can lead to gingivitis, which is where I was headed due to the inflammation of my gums. It could have developed into a further periodontal condition, and a much more serious infection that could cause tooth loss. I'm fortunate I caught the wave and changed my dental hygiene before reaching a place of no return.

When I returned to dental care, Mary was my first hygienist for a good fifteen years. I recall spitting in the bowl after a cleaning and seeing chunks of my gum along with blood. I know that's gross to admit, but I didn't know back then that wasn't good. When Mary retired, I went to a new dental group because the dentist at Mary's office told me I needed a root canal.

In case you don't know, I'm terrified of needles. Dr. Mark was in the process of scheduling my procedure, but I abruptly stopped him and asked if he could prescribe Xanax because I was terrified—and a little "sleepy gas would be nice too." To my benefit, he didn't do such things and referred me to sedation dentistry, and my dental life took a drastic turn. It also turned out I didn't need a root canal, just a little filing for my bite.

Did you know that infections that start in your mouth have been linked to such complications and disease such as:

❖ Asthma
❖ Arthritis
❖ Stroke
❖ Respiratory problems
❖ Premature births
❖ Low-birth-weight babies
❖ Coronary artery disease.

My mom had a stroke at the age of 62, a few years younger than I, and passed away four years later. She was paralyzed the entire time, confined to a bed with her only escape using a bed lift to change her sheets. No, I wasn't going there—nor should you.

As you can see, basic grooming is crucial to the changes you can make with the fundamental 101 basket of tricks. Eat well, don't smoke, and get into the habit of brushing your teeth twice a day, using a good mouthwash to eliminate lingering bacteria.

And to take a step further, let's peek at your connection to nature and your aging process, which can catapult you into a whole new sphere of anti-aging—naturally. Hanging out in nature is better than just about anything you can do for your health, with the exception of movement, which we'll discuss in the upcoming chapters. But for now, we lean into aligning with nature in Chapter 15.

Personal Inventory Questions

1. *Whether you think you can, or you think you can't, you're right,* says Henry Ford. What do you think? Do you believe you can work basic grooming into a lifelong habit of changes to benefit you?

2. Think of this chapter as a basket of tricks that will lead to youthful appearance and behavior — naturally. Do you believe this is possible?

3. What challenges do you have with your basic grooming? What has gotten in your way?

4. Gigi looked on every dating site and found one frog after another, but no prince. Have you run into difficulty finding a life partner? If so, examine what you're looking for, and if you, yourself, are presenting that in your hunt.

5. Marla, a nurse practitioner, met Roger; a dashing cardiologist with dimples the size of grapes and perfect, all-white teeth to go with them. The only issue was he licked his fingers when he ate. Have you passed on a significant other based on a habit that was annoying to you? If not, do you wish you had passed?

6. Sally was every man's dream, but she often skipped brushing her teeth and wasn't interested in flossing or whitening them, but John couldn't overlook this one small detail in their otherwise perfect relationship. What do you think? Was that harsh? Do you have a "Sally" in your life?

7. Betty didn't believe in shaving, which she felt wasn't natural. This caused a break-up with Peter.

What were you thinking when you read that section? Was Peter too harsh?

8. Simply put, washing and bathing are the most important ways to maintain good health and protect us from infections, illnesses, and such. What does your bathing ritual look like? What was your takeaway from Jeb's experience of turning his life around merely by returning to taking care of himself?

9. Dental work can be costly, not to mention painful, but not maintaining teeth can age a person considerably. What are your dental maintenance habits? What could you improve?

10. Do you believe skipping dental care can lead you to miss the diagnosis of such complications as heart disease, diabetes, asthma, eating disorder damage, etc.? Looking at your family history and your own grooming habits, do you feel you have medical complications that were overlooked?

Chapter 15

Earthing

Give the world the best you have, and it may
never be enough.
Give the world your best, anyway.
~Mother Teresa

Many of us never feel good enough, or that we've tried hard enough, so words such as Mother Teresa's, *Give the world the best you have, and it may never be enough,* couldn't ring more true, but when she goes on to say, *"Give the world your best, anyway."* her advice stings. For some of us, the thought circles back to our not being good enough.

When do we throw in the towel and give up? Never. We have to rise from every fall and power on because that's what survival is all about — though doing just that may be hard.

"As we look back and survey the terrain to determine where we've been and where we are in relationship to where we're going, we clearly see that we could not have gotten where we are without coming the way we came," says Steven Covey in his *The 7 Habits of Highly Effective People: Powerful Lessons in Personal Change*.

We are who we are today because of all of our yesterdays, including every scrape and fall. Without our experiences, we'd not have come to know who we are, or know others for that matter. How can we give the world the best we have, even if it's not enough, but give the world our best, anyway, when we don't feel up to the task? Well, first, we have to start from our core self. And if we don't like that self, then that's where we begin.

To build the 'you' of today takes experiences, good and bad. And true, if you give the world the best you have, it may never be enough, but...as Mother Teresa, an Albanian Roman Catholic nun who spent much of her life in India and acquired Indian citizenship, says, *Give the world your best, anyway*. And who would know this better than Mother Teresa, who devoted her life to serving the poorest of the poor around the world.

Mother Teresa was the founder of the Order of the Missionaries of Charity, a congregation of women dedicated to helping the destitute. She was considered one of the 20th century's greatest

251

humanitarians. She was canonized as Saint Teresa of Calcutta in 2016. Her mission was to look after people *who nobody else was prepared to look after*. In 1952, she opened her first home for the dying, which allowed people to die with dignity (Biography Online).

> *It's not how much we do,*
> *but how much love we put in the doing.*
> *It's not how much we give,*
> *but how much love we put in the giving.*

> ~Mother Teresa, from *No Greater Love*

How much love can we put in the giving if we don't like ourselves? How do we carve out a liking of self? It seems we have to find a way to connect to self, which for me started by aligning with nature to become still and find self. Often, we're so caught up with our aging and how we look that we can't see past that to help others — with love and selflessness.

Mother Teresa was wise; she was connected to much more than looks or seeking kudos from society for good works. No, everything she did was from a selfless love for others. Most of us could never give as she did, but we can learn to connect to the simplicity of life as we search for wellbeing of body, mind, spirit, and self.

Connecting To the Earth

A few years back, my husband and I purchased 40 acres of the nearly 400 in Wisconsin that once belonged to my father and mother. I spent many years in my youth riding my albino Arabian horse, Pasha, through the landscape, but I was particularly attached to this 40 acres, as something about this spot called to me.

"The 40," also known as Southern Grace Lane, is a thick forest filled with northern white pine, spruce, Jack pine, wild flowers, and edible berries. Trees are crucial to the stabilization of the soil, and in slowing water runoff, thus preserving nature. They're left to grow, reaching up to the sky. Wisconsin forests are known for their hunting and fishing grounds, producing wildlife and recreational benefits as well as timber crops.

In these very parts, my heart lies, stemming from years back when I was a child in the Wautoma forests. The plush forests are known for cardinals, blue jays, crows, and streams where the dear and bear drink, sharing grounds with wild squirrel, chipmunks, raccoon, all while acorns and pinecones crunch underfoot while these creatures browse on raspberries, which run wild for the picking.

In my teenage years, I was insecure, hyper-focused on my body image, and saddled with quite the undiagnosed eating disorder. Early years, I wasn't about my body, in the sense that I felt I wasn't thin enough—especially in my formative years when I had no visible weight problem, though I'd eat enough sweets to warrant one.

The only place of peace where my mind shut down was out on the acres—one with Pasha. My time with her out there was a time of prayer and aligning to nature. The land was quiet, with the exception of Pasha snorting or swishing at flies with her tail as they buzzed about, and the crunch of pines needles when we powered through the forest. This was my serenity.

Something about the earth always called me. Even when I was a small child, I'd make my way into the woods across from the cottages on Big Silver Lake in Wautoma, Wisconsin. Sometimes I made my way in too deep and became disoriented and lost, but I never feared what might be out there. I felt safe.

Instead, I would spend countless hours daydreaming about what life would be like living among the animals in the woods. I imagined being free of traffic and noise, as we lived in Chicago, which was anything but quiet. I loved the sounds of the forest, a natural symphony created by the singing and calling of the birds and noise of the deer skidding off into the deeper parts of the woods when I startled mamma and fawn.

The land was a place of serenity, a connecting to something greater and more important. This was a place where I could feel the earth, trees, and all that nature could provide, filling my nose with heavenly scents of pine, grass, and earth. I felt centered.

A Taste of Earthing, Anyone?
Back in those early days I didn't know what I was doing had a name, that it's called *earthing*. Some great sages suggest in order to connect with ourselves, we

need to first connect to the earth. *Earthing* is considered one of the most important self-care practices we can do each day.

I found, out there in the woods with Pasha, and earlier in my formative years, that I could hear an inner wisdom telling me what I needed to do next. You could say I was connected to my higher source, the earth, and my inner source all rolled into one — I felt a sense of home and wholeness, which later became foreign to me when I was caught up in the pleasing of others for acceptance. When I was trapped by the idea of my body not being thin enough.

Mother Teresa didn't please others for attention and acceptance; no, her motivation for all she did was pure love of another, no matter the cost to her physically. She wasn't living in posh conditions and often didn't know where her next meal would come from. Her life was by no means a fancy, upper-class existence; pure giving to others was what sustained her.

My Grandmother Ruth loved horses and riding through the woods, to the point that she opened a riding ranch next to my great paternal Grandpa Al's resort, where the city folk came to vacation. This was the very place my mother met my musician father, the good-looking city slicker who served as entertainment for the guests. Those were happy times, though afterward, somehow, my grandmother, and perhaps my mom, lost their way due to life's occurrences.

After the death of my grandmother's husband (and mom's father), a grandpa I never met, in her mid-adult years, Ruth struggled with weight, and maybe even alcoholism. She left her riding ranch and nature, as she knew it — no longer being in touch with her best self. When she was elderly and lived in a nursing home run by the White Habit Nuns, however, I saw a complete positive turnaround with her. The nuns provided a lovely environment where she was well cared for.

At the nursing home, my grandma ate natural foods, had two lovebirds in a golden cage in her room, and enjoyed a lovely terrace where she could go outside. She loved the outdoors. She loved the sun; she'd tip her head back and smile as she felt the warm sun on her face.

I took so much from this grandma — the good and the bad. But her love of the earth, animals, and nature was the best gift she could give. I remember a time when I was barely 13, my sister Mickey and I rode all the way to Florida with our grandparents, one in their powder-blue Cadillac, and the other in a pink Cadillac, towing the last bits of their belongings since they were moving to Florida.

As we crossed the border line from Georgia to Florida, we stopped at the welcome station where we were treated to a glass of freshly squeezed Florida orange juice, cold and filled with pulp — a delicious memory. I was barefoot and free — walking across the grass to the facility. The great sages say putting our bare feet on the ground outside for ten to twenty minutes a day helps to reduce chronic inflammation, the primary cause of virtually all diseases.

When was the last time you went barefoot on the grass...or the earth? As a kid, I lived all summer, *every summer* barefoot. I felt liberated and connected to the earth. I've learned since that our skin serves as a conductor, and when we touch any part of our skin to the earth, free electrons—the most powerful antioxidants available—flow from the earth into our bodies.

I recall when I was just out of high school with no direction, confidence, or belief in me. I felt I couldn't actually go to college, because I believed I wasn't smart enough. I took a job at a lab called Shara Labs, where they made vitamins. I glued labels on the vitamin bottles.

One of the owner's uncles also worked there. His name, Irwin, comes to my mind, along with his personality. He was quiet, always seemed to be thinking. He wore crisp, pressed tan khaki pants with a hunter-green polo neatly bearing the company logo below the left shirt pocket. He always had on elegant brown shoes. One day I caught him outside by the tall pine trees, a type of tree that fills much of the woods in Wisconsin; he had one hand on one tree and the other on another tree.

I watched Irwin quietly for quite some time. When he opened his eyes and saw me gawking, he said, "You ought to try this. I'm connecting to the earth and the sky—through energy." I never forgot.

Hug a Tree

At first I thought Irwin a bit odd, but when I touched the trees I felt something—I felt the energy he spoke of. And the energy is not just in Wisconsin but anywhere and everywhere you find an outdoors and trees. Now, I, too, know the vibration of the earth when I'm up at my getaway place on the west coast of Florida, the very home my Grandmother Ruth and Grandfather Hale purchased all those years back when we were kids, where I'm the owner after my mom.

My mom planted tall palm trees in the back of the house with a water backdrop, the Gulf of Mexico. In the evening, I often stand with my arms outstretched, touching one tree with one hand and the other with my other hand while looking up at the stars in the evening. Each time it reminds me of Irwin, my grandmother, and my mom, all lovers of nature.

I came to know the earth was my safe place, believing in order to connect with ourselves we need to first connect to the earth—and for me that's an extension of God or my understanding of a higher source. Instead of worrying about wrinkles, body weight, and aging, when I'm outdoors I'm grounded. Every morning I walk with Grace or cycle in the vicinity of the Intercoastal Waterway or the beach to connect and stabilize—something I learned from Irwin.

Stephen Covey writes, *Some people say that you have to like yourself before you can like others.* Though he thought that this belief had merit, he went on to say that if you don't know yourself, if you can't control yourself, if you don't have mastery over yourself, it's very hard to like yourself, except in some short-term, psych-up, superficial way.

And for sure that's what this book is about, existing as our best authentic selves, without being plastic. To be our true self without the entire set of fake bells and whistles. This is no easy feat when we're bombarded with commercials, articles, and social media telling us if we don't tuck this or change that, we're not being our best self. And maybe we'll find some small truth in that as we saw in Chapter 14, Little Things Do Count—as the idea relates to grooming.

Yes, many of us never feel good enough, or that we've tried hard enough, so words such as Mother Teresa's: *Give the world the best you have, and it may never be enough* could not ring more true, but when she goes on to say, *"Give the world your best, anyway,"* we need to take these words and live by them. We are good enough, right now.

Let's present our best self going forward and give our time to others—be our best—and do it with love. Go hug a tree and feel the earth under your toes, experience nature's love—a connection to your spiritual self. And to that point, as we move on to Chapter 16, God and the Spiritual Self, we will come to understand the entire objective of reaching our inner self as it connects to that higher self.

Personal Inventory Questions

1. Mother Teresa's, *Give the world the best you have and it may never be enough* could not ring more true, but when she goes on to say, *"Give the world your best, anyway,"* it stings. Do you give the best you have and feel it's not good enough? And do you give it anyway? How would your life change if you lived these words?

2. "As we look back and survey the terrain to determine where we've been and where we are in relationship to where we're going, we clearly see that we could not have gotten where we are without coming the way we came (Steven Covey). Do you need to come from where you came to be your best self?

3. Mother Teresa was wise; she was connected to much more than looks or seeking kudos from society for good works. Does such a life fit with your internal message?

4. In my younger years I spent a great deal of time riding my horse, Pasha, out in the forests. It was a place I could find great peace and forget my body, appearance, and self. Where was your place as a kid? Where is it now?

5. My Grandmother Ruth loved horses and riding through the woods to the point she opened a riding ranch next to my uncle's resort where the city folk came to vacation. I always felt my grandmother was living her best life back then but lost her way. When do you feel you lived your

best life? Is it now? What would you need to find your best you?

6. Stephen Covey writes, *Some people say that you have to like yourself before you can like others.* But he also explains why some people may not like themselves. Do you like you? What might you need to do to arrive at that place?

7. Some great sages suggest in order to *connect* with ourselves, we need to first connect to the earth. *Earthing* is considered one of the most important self-care practices we can do each day. Are you the earthing type?

8. When was the last time you walked barefoot on the earth, sand, or in the grass? How did it make you feel?

9. I described Irwin, the tree toucher, who at first, I thought was a bit odd. But when I touched the trees I felt something—I felt the energy he spoke of. Have you ever touched the base of a tree and felt the energy?

10. Mother Teresa didn't please others for attention and acceptance; no, she was motivated by pure love Do you have pure love for another? For others, in general.

Chapter 16

God And The Spiritual Self

And the day came when
the risk to remain tight in a bud
Was more painful than
the risk it took to blossom.
~Anais Nin

Do you jump in the water and swim, or do you dip in your toe, and slowly, inch by inch, make your way to the actual immersion? Which is better? Sometimes diving in and taking the plunge works best to avoid the painful reintroduction of cold water to each subsequent body part.

In life, we may avoid taking risks for fear of the unknown, but as we grow older and wiser, we often take the plunge...*and the day came when the risk to remain tight in a bud was more painful than the risk it took to blossom.*

And we can blossom no matter our age. In fact, Joan Borysenko, PhD, author of *A Woman's Book Of Life: The Biology, Psychology, and Spirituality of the Feminine Life Cycle*, reports, "As studies demonstrate, the truth is that women continue to develop their strengths and actually bloom, rather than fade, with the advent of midlife." And I'll add to that...men do too. But can we do it alone? Where does spirituality step in? Where does God fit into this scenario?

Body, mind, spirit means that our *well-being* comes from not just physical health, but from mental and spiritual health as well. Mental health includes our emotional, psychological, and social well-being. This combination affects how we think, feel, and act. It's how we handle life's challenges, how we relate to others, and how we make choices.

The word "spiritual" points to a sense of completeness, to feeling connected with the earth and the universe. Spiritual health is achieved when you feel at peace with life — that self-actualization we discussed in the earlier chapters. You have spiritual health when you're able to find hope and comfort, in even the hardest of times.

The definition of God in most understandings is: "the creator and ruler of the universe and source of all moral authority — the Supreme Being" (definition from the *Oxford English Dictionary*. Merriam-Webster defines God as: "the supreme or ultimate reality, such as the Being perfect in power, wisdom, and goodness, who is worshipped (as in Judaism, Christianity, Islam, and Hinduism) as creator and ruler of the universe."

As I've labored to bring this book into existence, perhaps the most surprising revelation has been how little we individuals know of our spiritual selves, and how starved we are for information. We need a blend of healthy self in body, mind, *and* spirit — that is, we are all more than just our thoughts, and more than just our bodies — the real package is bigger than that — much bigger.

The whole self of body, mind, and spirit is the elixir needed to create the best you possible. Throughout the previous pages, we looked at the body and the mind and the spirit, but now I want to focus and look more closely at your belief in something higher and greater than your mortal self.

And you can call this higher source whatever you wish. We often become caught up in names such as God or Jesus, Elohim, Yahweh, Jehovah, or Adonai, but taking that as a definition may block you from your intimate connection, whatever you want to call it.

I'd like to think that everyone has a personal take on his or her own *Divine Source*, whether from Judaism, for instance, or through Buddhism, Sikhism, Christianity, or whatever reference point, perhaps combined with another particular spiritual training.

Regardless of *your* concept of Source, you can tap into your own heart and soul using the approach that fits your belief system best, to find an authentic foundation and open the door to a much deeper, more soulful experience of life — as you *heal from the inside out.*

Happiness Every Day

In the opening of *Every Day a Friday: How to Be Happier 7 Days a Week,* Joel Osteen shares a story about John, a ninety-two-year-old blind man, sharp as could be, who was preparing to move into a nursing home facility after the passing of his wife, Eleanor.

As John was about to tour the site, and his new room, he said, "I love it. I love it. I love it." Now mind you, John hadn't seen his room yet, nor the rest of the facility.

When questioned about this, he said, "No you don't have to show it to me. Whether I like my room or not doesn't depend on how the furniture is arranged. It depends on how my mind is arranged. Happiness is something you decide ahead of time."

These words speak volumes. What he said is deeper than the fact that this man didn't need to see his room to determine if he liked the room or not. His statement was about his mindset. He was centered.

How do we become centered? Can we do it alone, or do we need that connection to something greater than self? And that connection is a personal connection; as mentioned earlier, it's whatever is right for you. Often making the connection is about attitude — looking at the glass as half full, rather than half empty, or seeing the sun shinning, rather than the clouds closing in on you.

We need to see the smiles, not the frowns, the laughter, not the tears. If you believe this is going to be a great day, it most likely will be. On the other hand, if you believe the day is going to one of drudgery, it may be that. Set your mind—your tone for the day, and watch the miracles unfold.

In Susan Hill's *Dangerous Prayers, 50 Powerful Prayers That Changed the World*, she notes that when Johann Sebastian Bach composed each new piece, he wrote the letters JJ, short for J*esus* Juvo, or "Jesus help"—at the top of the page, and SDG, *Soli Deo Gloria*, at the bottom of the page for "the glory of God alone." His prayer was that whenever the music was played, it would point toward God.

Bach was setting his mind. He expected to start his music in God's prayer and end it there as well. Let's stretch that and start our day in God's prayer by setting our minds. John, about to move to perhaps an uncertain future, set his mind to a positive mindset, while Bach set his mind to start his composition in God's prayer and end in God's prayer.

How do you set your mind? Does it point toward God (or your understanding of a higher source) and end with for the glory of God alone? When you open your eyes on the day, what's your first thought? Do you know? Do you wake rested?

Sleep a Natural Medicine

Often we don't sleep enough, which not only ages us, but also leaves us discombobulated—confused. Sleep is crucial to our physical, mental, and spiritual health.

On a physical plane, our sleeping hours are a time to heal and repair our heart and blood vessels, not to mention that ongoing sleep deficiency puts us at risk of heart disease, kidney disease, high blood pressure, diabetes, and stroke. And hey, lack of sleep contributes to aging poorly—bags under the eyes and less pep and concentration.

Did you know a lack of quality sleep also weakens the skin's ability to repair itself at night and could cause you to actually look older? And scarier still is that researchers have discovered just a single night of insufficient sleep can make an older adults' cells age more quickly.

On a spiritual level, our sleep hours are a time to rest the mind—escape the stress of the day. The Bible says on the seventh day God rested, and later commanded we do the same. And if God built sleep into our life, it must be super important. And heck, even Jesus slept, just the way we do. Think of sleep as a gift to replenish our bodily health and to give us the much-needed rest from our waking hours.

Sleep time is an opportunity to shut down from the worries of the day—to hand them over or shelf them so peace and security can take over. I've found my sleeping hours are my best time to come up with strategies and creative ideas—perhaps imparted to me directly from the Divine. Some say sleep is an opportunity to encounter the Holy Spirit through prophetic dreams and songs in the night...as we read repeatedly in the Bible.

Some say they have bad dreams, or encounters of a demonic sort, or nightmares; perhaps this is an indication that such folks are not on course with their best life. Perhaps it's a hint that change is needed. If you engage in drugs, alcohol, or poor quality foods — or maybe feel guilt about something you've done, or didn't do, such causes could impact the quality of your sleep.

Perhaps sleep is an opportunity to cleanse from these bad habits or concerns. In Psalms 127:2 it says: *Even when awake in the night hours, our reflections can be full of God's grace*, rather than turmoil. The Bible also says that rising early, and retiring late is unwise. I'll admit I'm guilty of this, as I tend to go to bed close to midnight and wake up around 6:15 daily. I don't need an alarm. My body simply requires only this much sleep, no matter where I am or in what time zone or country I need no more than six and a half hours of sleep. And I'm good, not tired, but clear minded until close to midnight, and then I'm done.

And face it, if we aren't well rested, we'll not be fully awake and engaged during the day, but rather wanting only to make our way through the day. Doesn't the idea of waking rested to begin our new day in the grace of God, or whatever you believe in, much better than to wake in worry, dreading what's ahead.

Perhaps starting the day in prayer and ending in prayer is the ticket to peace and tranquility. Of course, prayer is personal and individual. So often, we make prayer — a simple connection to our higher self —

complicated. It doesn't have to be. It can be a conversation with your understanding of deity.

The Bible, James 5:15, reads, "The prayer of a righteous person is powerful and effective." What makes prayer powerful is to pray because you want to — because you long for that connection to carry you during tough times. For many, prayer takes them out of the worry and into a place of peace.

For me, prayer is something I learned early in my childhood, and to date I'm grateful as it has kept me afloat through rough times knowing, *this too shall pass.*

Forgiveness Will Set You Free

Maybe you are living life with anger over something that happened to you or someone who did you wrong. The Dalai Lama, in *The Wisdom of Forgiveness: Intimate Conversations and Journeys,* says forgiving your enemies can make a big difference in your spiritual progress. He says forgiveness is crucial, that it's one of the most important spiritual steps, that it can change your life. Forgiveness is for our own growth and happiness.

When we hold on to hurt, pain, resentment, and anger it harms us far more than it harms the person who did us wrong. Learning to forgive will free us to live in the present — *Let go...let God.* Holding onto anger, regret, hatred, or resentment toward another is to give our power to that person.

Stephen R. Covey in *The 7 Habits of Highly Effective People* looks at the difference between proactive and reactive individuals. The proactive person focuses energy on the things they can do something about. The nature of their energy is positive and magnifying. The reactive person, on the other hand, focuses their energy on blaming and accusing attitudes, reactive language, and increased feelings of victimization.

Put this type of knee-jerk response into a forgiveness perspective and imagine what the proactive person versus the reactive person would do. For sure the proactive individual is going to let go...and let God—while the reactive person is going to go down the "why me" road filled with anger and rage—not forgiveness. And for certain, forgiveness will set you free. It's the opposite of what you might think.

Perhaps your thought is that forgiveness shows weakness rather than strength. But who suffers when you hold onto victimhood and the blame game? Without a doubt the reactive person is not going to be free. Forgiveness lightens the burden for the forgiver, regardless of what harm the other person did.

Richard Carlson in *You Can Be Happy No Matter What: Five Principles Your Therapist Never Told You* opens his book with: "Happiness! It's something that all of us want but that few of us ever achieve. It is characterized by feelings of gratitude, inner peace, satisfaction, and affection for ourselves and for others." He goes on to say, "Our most natural state of mind is one of contentment and joy."

Wow, our most natural state of mind is one of contentment and joy. Natural is a God-given gift, something we're all entitled to. But how can we arrive at that happy place if we're filled with anger and blame and unwilling to forgive. Who can cast that first stone? You know, let him who is without sin cast the first stone. Or in the old proverb, people who live in glass houses shouldn't throw stones. Nobody is perfect.

During the pandemic, which started while I was midway through writing this book and continues as the book comes to a close, many sad stories made the rounds. Believing a kind and loving God would allow such a pandemic to affect the entire world is difficult. Has he? Beth Moore in *Believing God* says, "We somehow want to neatly package God and make everything about Him explainable. We decide that what's not explainable is not plausible. We make God behave and fit into our textbooks."

Well, the Higher Source, whom some of us call God, just doesn't work that way. We can't bend and force our belief system to behave the way we want it to. As we are seeking our best life, our fresh, youthful side, life happens, and all that we try to make happen can unravel.

But if we believe better days are coming or a lesson can be learned from all of this, everything we see in front of us becomes okay. My dad prayed all the way to his last breath. Though his mind wasn't always intact, he never lost his connection—this I treasure as I'm moving through my own last act in this life.

Some of us are tearing down statues from different belief systems, as restlessness ensues. And to

271

some, God or any belief, whether organized religion or spiritual or a combination of the two, is just not cool.

So health and a healthy lifestyle in some situations has been tossed to the side during these tough times, or just in general times. Several of my patients as of late—eight to be exact—ended up in a treatment facility for alcoholism, eating disorder, and drug overdose. Our path doesn't have to take this route. We can turn to a higher energy of our liking, and life becomes a whole lot easier. As we move on to Chapter 17, you can *imagine* your later life into reality. This chapter is going to show you how to do that through guided imagery with a mix of meditation. The goal is to carry you to and through the future, to establish the later years in your now present years.

Personal Inventory Questions

1. Do you jump in the water and swim, or do you dip in your toe, and slowly, inch by inch, make your way to the actual immersion? Which is better?
2. Anais Nin says, *And the day came when the risk to remain tight in a bud was more painful than the risk it took to blossom.* How have you blossomed?
3. Body, mind, spirit means that our *well-being* comes from not just physical health, but from mental and spiritual health as well. How is your mental health? How is your spiritual health?
4. The definition of God, in most understandings, is the creator and ruler of the universe and source of

all moral authority, the Supreme Being (Definitions from *Oxford English Dictionary*). How do you define your understanding of God?

5. In the opening of *Every Day a Friday: How to Be Happier 7 Days a Week,* Joel Osteen shares a story about John, a ninety-two-year-old blind man, sharp as could be, who was about to move into a nursing home after the passing of his wife, Eleanor. Before John ever saw his new room, he said, "I love it. I love it. I love it." How did his positive attitude — his mindset — match yours?

6. When Johann Sebastian Bach composed each new piece, he wrote the letters JJ, short for *Jesus Juvo,* or "Jesus help" — at the top of the page, and SDG, *Soli Deo Gloria*, at the bottom of the page for "the glory of God alone." His prayer was that whenever the music was played, it would point toward God. What is your God practice?

7. Often, we don't sleep enough, which not only ages us, but also leaves us discombobulated — confused. How much sleep do you get? Is it leaving you discombobulated, or do you wake fresh?

8. For many, prayer takes them out of worry and into a place of peace. Do you have a prayer practice? Do you believe in the power of prayer? How has prayer played in your life?

9. Maybe you're living with anger over something that happened to you, or toward someone who did you wrong. The Dalai Lama, in *The Wisdom of Forgiveness: Intimate Conversations and Journeys,* says to forgive, that to forgive your enemies can

make a difference in your spiritual progress. What do you think — can forgiving your enemy make a difference to you on your spiritual journey?

10. Richard Carlson, PhD, in his *You Can Be Happy No Matter What: Five Principles Your Therapist Never Told You* opens the book with: "Happiness! It's something that all of us want but that few of us ever achieve." Are you happy — truly happy?

Chapter 17

Imagine Your Later Years into Reality

To accomplish great things,
we must not only act,
but also dream; not only plan,
but also believe.
~Anatole France

When we not only act, but also dream, not only plan, but also believe, then we will see the magic happen, the dreams blossom into fruition. A great starting place is to look at our later years with a fresh pair of eyes. This chapter is going to show you how to do that through guided imagery with a mix of meditation. The goal is to carry you to and through the future, to establish the later years in your now present years.

In order to create change, to look at our lives through a revised perception, we need to believe that having a new vision of the future is possible. And sometimes, a little nudge is in order to make that adjusted, brighter picture come to life. In my office, self-hypnosis is one of the powerful tools I offer that many patients take advantage of. But, since you're over wherever you are, reading, and I'm here—somewhere—rather than hypnosis, we're going to put together a perfect anti-aging guided imagery meditation script for you to adapt and record for your own personal use.

Your Thoughts Are Powerful

The human mind is powerful, and putting together words of your choice to embed can take on a life of its own—creating potent change.

So, what is guided imagery? Well, the process has been called by many different names, including: guided meditation, visualization, mental rehearsal, and guided self-hypnosis. Rather than becoming caught up in the name, think of guided imagery as a powerful technique that focuses our imagination in a proactive, positive way.

Personally, I like to think of guided imagery meditation as a way for us to tap into the five basic senses: sight, hearing, touch, taste, and smell, so that we can send information to the brain to assist us in perceiving and understanding the world around us.

As guided imagery personally relates to you, the individual conducting the guided imagery, it can combat the obsessive, nagging aging dialogue in your head.

The script provided here is yours to change any way you see fit. I'm giving you loose guidance that *you* will tighten, inserting your personal wants and needs. If you have a smartphone, simply press 'record,' and slowly read the script. If you don't have a phone, dig out your old recorder of whatever type and record.

Make your recording in a soft tone...almost a whisper. If you want, put some music in the background to set the tone. The cool thing is this recording is for your ears only, so go for it and don't be hypercritical. Personally I'd use ear buds so that the reading goes directly into your ear, which gives it a richer sound, without critics asking you what you're doing, because they can't hear you.

If you don't want to hear your voice, then use software to read the script to you. Once it's set it's yours to listen to any time you want. I use a program called Natural Reader when I want something read to me. Natural Reader is software that allows you to listen to any text on your computer or phone.

With Natural Reader, you can actually listen to your emails, web news, and other reading materials, but I use it strictly for my manuscripts, or if I'm endorsing someone's book and I have to read the manuscript. This program allows me to listen while

I'm getting ready for work, cleaning house, or taking my morning walks. It's a fabulous time saver.

Natural Reader can convert any written text such as in MS Word, Webpage, PDF format, and emails into spoken words with Microsoft voices. I do use the version for which I paid a small one-time fee to pick the voice I wanted. I found a woman's voice very similar to mine.

For guided imagery and meditation purposes, you can slow down the voice, way down, so that you can hear each word and meditate on it. The result is awesome! It's like going to someone for guided imagery, but you're in the comfort of your own home. Now don't do this while driving. I do it on my walks but what I'm doing isn't meditation, yet rather listening to chapters from my books.

If you don't like your voice, or you feel goofy using your own voice, then write out your script to your liking, and use a program that can read it to you. When my manuscripts are ready for edits, I listen to each chapter through Natural Reader while I'm walking. I hear mistakes my eyes don't catch, which gives me the opportunity to read and correct before sending it off to my amazing editor.

Simply type into Google the words 'Natural Reader,' and you'll see a free version pop up. From there, all you have to do is download the program on a device of your choice. As I mentioned, I use my phone but you can use whatever you're comfortable with.

So Let's Begin:

Before starting, let's go over some simple, basic actions you might want to take to set your mindset. First, you always want to make sure you're in a comfortable room where you'll not be interrupted or disturbed. Turn off your phone(s) — the vibration feature too. If you have pets that might jump on you, perhaps moving them out of the room would be a good idea. Find a comfortable chair or place a mat on the floor, or even lie down on your couch or bed. All good. Keep it simple. Keep it fun.

The goal is to use *your* guided imagery meditation to visualize positive actions, changes, and/or accomplishments, no matter your age. Age is just a number and doesn't define you. Ask yourself questions such as: What do I want to change? What accomplishments are calling me? Visualize what you want and set it in action. When you see it and believe it, and act as if you are it, you're well on your way.

Now you might be thinking, *Oh but I'm too old for change*, or *I don't have money*, or *I can't do that — it's too late*. No, stop that. In order for any type of guided imagery to take hold, you must believe it is so. The great thing about the subconscious mind is that it doesn't know the difference between real and pretend. So go for it. Think big.

Of course before you enter any hypnotic or relaxed state, make sure you're not driving, as you will be in a dream-like kind of mind. You may be thinking, *Oh boy what if I don't come out of it*. Trust me, you will. And your script is going to bring you back to a conscious state from the wording you record. If you fall asleep, no worries, you'll still derive what you need…and have a nap, too.

Begin the process with a few slow, deep breaths in through your nose and out through your mouth, letting your whole body relax. When I'm working with a patient, I have them do cycle breathing in which they breathe in slowly to the count of four, then hold their breath to the count of four, and then exhale to the count of four.

Again, you can choose to do your guided imagery in a chair or lying on a mat or even in your bed if you like. Now, though I've set down a script below, you can put your own twist on it, filling the blanks as they make sense to you.

For example, where I say use your imagination, and picture yourself walking slowly along the shoreline with the ocean as your backdrop, you may prefer to walk along a path through the woods with fall leaves in full orange and red array, or you may want to hike up a mountainside. So take the script, adjust, and then record, which allows you to go for the imagery ride, listening to your own voice guiding your journey.

Remember, the idea is to follow your own imagination, so the script is loosely set. Make sure to allow for long pauses, so you can let your imagination roam. Also, consider playing soft classical music, or spa radio, or beach and natural sounds softly in the background. Don't pick anything with lyrics or commercials because that will pull you out of your imagery.

Read through the script a few times to work out the kinks before recording. Remember the *I* in the script is *you,* not me the writer. You might want to change up the words or scenery, which is perfect, as this is your ride, solely for you. You'll note that I repeat words in my sample script, which is intentional. You need to keep reinforcing what you want to experience.

At first, you might feel wonky listening to your own voice, but that will change in time. Your recording won't sound goofy at all once you become used to it. You might, in fact, grow to love the sound of your own voice.

Now that you're in your comfortable spot, you will play your recorded reading.

Start Your Recording

Begin to speak from this point on... Remember to speak slowly and ease yourself into the relaxed state...

. . . .

It's time, time for you to sit quietly, close your eyes, and begin to relax. Let yourself begin to relax and feel calm, with peace of mind. Just feel yourself at ease—tranquil, at peace, relaxed.

Take in a long, slow, breath now, all the way in, to the count of four... Hold it to the count of four... And then release to the count of four. With each breath, as you exhale, this calmness becomes stronger and stronger, spreading all the way from your head

281

down to your toes, from top to bottom, inside out and outside in, immersing you into an ocean of calm.

Relax your body by releasing any areas of tension... Allow your arms to go limp...then your legs... Feel the calmness...an ocean of calmness... That's right. Feel your arms and legs becoming loose and relaxed. Now, relax your neck and back by relaxing your spine... Let go... Relax all your muscles now... all the way from your head, down your neck...along each vertebra...to the tip of your spine.

Smell the sweet, salty ocean air. Hear the sounds of the waves crashing on the shoreline. Imagine your bare feet sinking into the warm, wet sand along the ocean with the cool saltwater lapping up to your ankles. Feel the soft breeze... Be there...

Can you notice how light and free you feel? See your young self as you push forward.

Take another deep breath... Breathe deeply into your diaphragm, drawing the air fully into your lungs... Hold it... And release the air with a whooshing sound... And you can be pleased. Everything you imagine to be so, becomes so.

See yourself full of energy, bright, clear minded...strong.

Breathe in again, slowly... Pause for a moment... And as you let out the breath, feel all the tensions leaving, leaving your body — going out of you, out of your body. You feel at peace, calm, and at ease. All bothers, worries, anxieties, just fading away, just fading away. Gone, gone far away.

There's lots of time. You have lots of time...so much time... Feel your mind at peace, calm, at peace, relaxed and at ease... Your mind becomes calm, your mind and body are at ease, peaceful and relaxed.

You have now become *so* deeply relaxed...*so* deeply asleep...that your mind has become *very* sensitive...very receptive to what I say...that *everything* I put into your mind...will sink *very* deeply into the unconscious part of your mind...and will cause so deep and lasting an impression there...that nothing will eradicate it.

Consequently...these things that I put into your unconscious mind...will begin to exercise a greater and greater influence over the way you feel...over the way you behave. You are more and more ready to retain those ideas that I will give you, as you will let them go deep into the back of your mind, and you will use them as you wish throughout your life.

And...because these things will remain firmly embedded in the unconscious mind, every day, beginning now, you'll feel this way, calm, and at peace, strong and sturdy...while you're interacting, while you're working, while you're doing whatever you need to do, you'll still feel peaceful, calm, and at ease. You will have energy...see your young self...

You are now *so very deeply asleep*...that *everything* I tell you that is going to happen to you for your own good will happen...*exactly* as I tell you. And every feeling...I tell you that you will experience...you *will* experience...*exactly* as I tell you. And these same things will continue to happen to you...every day...just as strongly....just as surely...just as powerfully...when you are out and about or when you are here in this room.

Think for a moment about your body. No matter the shape or size, your body is magnificent and beautiful. Your body is composed of individual cells, which work together in harmony to keep you at your very best. The you now is the future you as you imagine it to be.

You are able to enjoy life now, with peace of mind, at peace with the universe, a feeling of peace and tranquility. A *knowing* you can set out to do what you really want to do. Nothing is stopping you. You have strength; the changes you want occur...it's all yours.

And you have a feeling that it's so good to be alive with peace of mind. At peace, you are at peace with everyone around you, relaxed and calm and at ease, and enjoying every moment of living. Starting now, a feeling of underlying happiness and peace of mind can be yours, can be with everyone in the universe, a feeling of peace and tranquility.

And a feeling is yours that being alive with peace of mind is very good. At peace with everyone around you, especially with yourself, relaxed and calm and at ease, and enjoying every moment of living from now going forward.

Starting now, a feeling of underlying happiness, and peace of mind can be with you, can be with everyone in the universe, because we create it ourselves, as we *let* our mind be calm and relaxed.

As you continue to walk the shoreline, hear the birds, smell the ocean, and feel the breeze, and as you become calmer and more relaxed, you *feel* a kind of underlying energy. The relaxation and calmness fits in with energy, vitality, being fully alive, in all times and in all situations.

During this sleep state, you will feel more and more *alert*. Starting now, you'll *feel* calmer and calmer, at ease, and at peace, feeling so good to be alive. You are now so *very deeply asleep...* You are going to feel physically *stronger* and more fit in every way. You will feel more alert...more wide awake...more energetic, more youthful.

So good to be vibrant, energetic, vital, healthy and strong...so alive and vibrant, able to *flow* with everything around you, every day, and to enjoy every day, more and more, to enjoy every aspect of every day, as you *feel* peaceful, and calm, *and at ease*, with energy, with vitality, feeling the strength and energy in your being, feeling the flowing and vibrations and energetic flow of your life.

Take another deep breath...in...and out...become even more and more relaxed with each breath...feel your body giving up all the tension...becoming relaxed...and calm...peaceful...as though you're floating. With each breath as you exhale, this calmness becomes stronger and stronger, spreading all the way from your head down to your toes, from top to bottom, inside out and outside in, immersing you in an ocean of calmness.

An ocean of calmness…that's right…and as that continues, peace and serenity are taking you over, inside and outside, thus putting your mind and body in sync with each other. Your body is strong…it carries you wherever you need to go….it doesn't let you down…*your* body is strong…*feel it…own it…be it.*

I want to remind you of something that you probably already know, which is you feel good…*you know*…deep inside…everything is good…I would like you to discover your inner dreams, your bliss…see it in your mind.

With peace of mind, calm, and remaining at ease, being able to look out at every part of the universe, at *every* person around you, at *every* flower smelling the sweet scent…*feeling* the strength of the tree and spry as a vine climbing up the trunk…*feel* the soft warm breeze, and now embrace the child in you, and in a new way, with a freshness, and wonder, and awe of a little child.

You begin now to see the world again as you once did when you were a small child…filled with wonder…wide eyed and filled with excitement and awe. And…you can regain that capacity again to see and appreciate everything freshly, and naively, in a simple way as you can begin once again to see things anew, fresh, wonderful, clean.

Now you can begin to look at every sunrise as if it's the first sunrise you've ever seen, and every sunset with more to come, and you will see the colors, and the wonder, and the beauty surrounding you *again*, as if it's the first time you're ever seen it.

Starting now, every bird that you see will seem as if you've never seen a bird before, as if you're a new child, and you're *beginning again* to look with wonder and amazement at the world around you. You *see* every bird, you hear every bird...in a *new* way, and every tree, and the leaves on the tree, and the seeds on the tree, and the bark on the tree, and the green leaves and the sun shinning, and the grass around you, you'll be able to see it all in a new way, fresh, *with wonder and awe.*

As you gain the capacity to appreciate everything as you once did, everything that's become stale over the years will no longer be stale for you...as you become aware again that we can be the way we were once, looking at each thing as miraculous, as beautiful, as wonderful *as the first time* we ever saw them, when we were children.

With this *new* way of looking at life, you'll find every day that *your* energy *will* increase, and you'll find *every day* that your energy *will* increase and you'll *feel* so healthy, and you feel healthy and free, you'll feel free from all the tensions...tensions will leave.

From this day on, you'll begin to live *fully*, moment by moment, every day. You'll gain so much out of every day, more and more, starting now, every day, every hour, every second, you will become more and *more exciting, full, enthralling, amazing.* You *will* become more and more aware of the wonders of your being, yourself, the earth, and everything around you.

The child in you *will* emerge. You'll again remember how to play and how to have fun, how to laugh...how to smile...by your own creativity and imagination, using your own ingenuity, able to regain your lost spontaneity, your naturalness, your freshness — it will come out and you will feel at ease with it.

As you think about this, it's becoming part of you, it *is* you. You will be less and less worried about the future, problems of the future, dangers of the future, which will never come to pass anyway. Today is your new beginning. The child in you awakens with open eyes, open heart, and a new wave of creativity.

Soon...soon...soon it will be time to come back into the room, taking with you all of your new treasures, as they are yours. I'm going to count up from one to five and at the count of five you will open your eyes, coming back into the room, feeling fresh and whole.

One...you are with peace of mind, calm, and at ease, being able to look out at every part of the universe with new eyes. Two...every person around you, every flower and every tree and every plant...the grass and children you see with fresh eyes and fresh heart. Three...you are feeling closer and closer to the room, ready to take on your day with energy and vitality. Four...you're starting to feel your toes, legs, and the surroundings of the room. Five...open your eyes. It's time to open your eyes...

....

Now, at this point, you will feel refreshed and renewed. I'd sit with it for a while, reacquainting yourself with the room, your body, and your surroundings before getting up. Don't spend time thinking about the words or what you did in your conscious mind. Just let this fresh feeling take hold and do its thing and the change will take hold. The change is subtle yet pronounced.

You have much to look forward to. And with this new you, let's move on to Chapter 18, Something to Look Forward To. Life is brief, a blink of the eye, so don't waste a minute fretting about your time being over, when as long as you have breath in you, your opportunities still beckon.

Personal Inventory Questions

1. When we not only act but also dream, and we not only plan but we also believe, then you will see the magic happen, the dreams come into fruition. Do you believe dreams can come into fruition?

2. In order to create change or to look at things through fresh eyes, we need to believe that it's possible. And to start that process we have not only to believe dreams are possible, but also to create the dream. What is your dream?

3. Guided imagery meditation is not mumbo jumbo, it's actually quite powerful and can lead to great change. Have you ever done guided imagery with a dash of meditation before? What was the experience like?

4. If you've never done guided imagery meditation before, why not? Do you have a belief system that

tells you it's not okay? Where does this idea stem from?

5. The idea with guided imagery meditation is for us to tap into our organs associated with each sense: sight, hearing, touch, taste, and smell. Which of your senses is the strongest? Take that sense and plug more of it into your script.

6. Some people have a tough time hearing their own voice. Do you? What about your voice do you love? What don't you like? How will your reaction to your voice impact your recording process?

7. As you read through the guided imagery meditation script, what was your initial thought? Did you see areas you wanted to change? Did you change those areas to make the script fit for you?

8. Once you recorded your script, how did you feel? Did you feel giddy and hopeful, or silly and childlike? Either way, you are tapping into your deeper child self.

9. Remember the idea is to follow your own imagination, so the script is loosely set. Make sure to take long pauses so you can use your imagination. Did you consider playing music in the background? If so, how did that work for you?

10. Now that you've completed the exercise, think about making another script taking what you need from the one provided but truly making it your own. How does that idea strike you?

Chapter 18

Something To Look Forward To

It is never too late
to be what you might have been.
~George Eliot

It is never ever too late to be what you might have been. Okay, if you want to be a great speed runner in the Olympics, and you're nearing eighty years of age, you might not make it. But you can be a runner, and you can compete in your age category.

It's never too late. Don't avoid the things you really want to do, not now, not ever. Life is brief, a blink of the eye, so don't waste a minute fretting about your time being over, when as long as you have breath in you, your opportunities still beckon. You have much to look forward to.

I have many writer friends, too many to count, and they range from young adults to the elderly well in their eighties. They're going strong in their quest to write their stories, whether the great novel, or a non-fiction, wise piece of information. All good. And I think of my friends who are college professors in their seventies and eighties and are working—working strong. Don't let the numbers define you, or describe what you're capable of accomplishing.

You're Never Too Late

My Great Great Aunt Mary Starks made her way to Fairbanks, Alaska in 1943, leaving her family newspaper business where she was a journalist. In 1946, she enlisted in the military to write publicity releases at Ladd Army Air Force Base near Fairbanks. She was thirty-seven years old at a time when women weren't welcomed in the military, and she was pushing past the age of enlistment. She charged forward, even when others told her that her ambition was an impossible dream. In 1948, President Truman enabled a permanent presence of women in the military. Great Great Aunt Mary Starks made her new career happen though all odds were against her as a woman, and at thirty-seven years old.

Then Aunt Mary continued to forge ahead after she left Alaska, making her way back to Berlin, Wisconsin, her hometown. She was quoted as saying, "Once a newspaper reporter, always a newspaper reporter," when she started to write and edit a newsletter at the Berlin Memorial Hospital Nursing

Home. She was ninety-two, and continued until her passing a few months short of one-hundred years of age.

Never give up on your dreams...not now, not ever.

When I was nineteen years old, I stumbled upon *Your Erroneous Zones*, written by Dr. Wayne Dyer. I read those pages with a hunger, as if I'd never had such a meal. And perhaps I'd never had. His wise words gave me, an awkward nineteen-year-old, overweight, binge-eating bulimic, permission to take charge of myself and power through all of life's adversities. Maybe you, too, need permission to seize authority in your life. Take the leap and dream big.

From listening to Dr. Dyer's talks, reading his books, and speaking to him personally on his weekly talk show on Hay House Radio back in 2015, I learned his 213-page book was written in a single weekend at a hotel in Ft. Lauderdale, Florida during a turning point in his life. I was at a turning point as well when I first happened upon this lifesaving book in 1976.

I'm grateful I was able to tell Dr. Dyer during our lengthy talk how he was a light in my life. I, too, had been at one of my lowest points, and each word on the pages of *Your Erroneous Zones* ignited hope and inspiration that I'd not felt since I was a small child. He and I discussed books and book publishing, and my then manuscript, *Release Your Obsession with Food: Heal from the Inside Out*. (Here I am on book four in this series.)

We spoke of addictions and recovery, something we both had accomplished. We discussed how recovery had everything to do with self-love and wasn't about the viewpoints of others—the very words I'd read in his first book back in 1976. Again, I was at another turning point in my life.

Dr. Dyer passed away in 2015, a few short months after our talk.

Carve Out Your Dream

We can look forward to our future and carve out our dreams, something I began to practice from those early days in 1976 and continue to work on today. Making peace with our pasts and tuning to new dreams to look forward to is a tough one for most of us to grasp, including and especially those coming hard upon the later acts in our lives.

You can make excuses that you missed your chance, and you have nothing to look forward to, or you can create your vision of what you want to do with the time remaining. But the time is going to go by, anyway, so you might as well make it count for something. We all have the ability to take charge of ourselves and plan. Listen to Dr. Wayne Dyer in his first book, *Your Erroneous Zones*:

The next time you are contemplating a decision in which you are debating whether or not to take charge of yourself, to make your own choice, ask yourself an important question, "How long am I going to be dead?" With that eternal perspective, you can now make your own choice and leave the worrying, the fears, the question of whether you can afford it and the guilt to those who are going to be alive forever.

As harsh as that may sound, when you're dead, your span here on earth school is complete (unless we have such a thing as reincarnation, or do-overs). However, we have great and rewarding surprises ahead of us as long as we have breath. Society has a way of dictating what we should or shouldn't be doing at a certain age, but such opinions aren't necessarily true.

My father opened an additional music store when he was in his eighties, signing an extended lease with the expectation he'd be here and continue to run it, and he did. The business was only recently closed a few years *after* his passing at ninety-one.

Wendy, a flashy seventy-something who just finished writing her first novel, joined a group of savvy self-thinkers in a positive group forum, and opened a new travel business. And then I recall Anthony, who retired from a high profile position in Homeland Security, purchased a large piece of land, and opened a recreational hunting ground equipped with cabins. He dug a spring-fed lake and incorporated fun activities for the campers at the age of sixty-two.

Over the twenty-three years in my psychotherapy practice, I've asked patients, " Are you living your best life?" and "How's it working for you?" And most of the time the answer has been, "No, I'm not living my best life — and it's not working for me."

And by best life, I'm not *only* referring to a career choice, I'm looking at living life to the fullest, like the trip to Europe that you always dreamed of taking. Or maybe you always wanted to live in Hawaii but were afraid to move. Perhaps you always wanted to learn the piano, but you were told that at a certain age you can't learn to play an instrument. Rubbish. You *can* do what you always dreamed to do. You can.

Okay, why aren't you living your life with purpose—and starting with something you might look forward to? I gathered in my arsenal of notes and memories all the excuses I've heard as to why someone has nothing to look forward to. And with the excuses, come the parenthetical statements representing reasoning that justifies the pre-set logic.

Nothing to Look Forward To List
I have nothing to look forward to because:

1. *I'm too old* ("I missed my opportunity and now it's too late—I should have thought about this when I was younger and had more time").
2. *I'm broke* ("I didn't save for my golden years and now I'm paying the price").
3. *I'm depressed* ("I'm very sad and have no energy to create what's missing in my life").
4. *I'm not healthy* ("I have too many aches and pains to look forward to much").
5. *I'm so tired* ("I have no energy to start something new").

6. *What's the point?* ("Nothing ever works for me so why try now").

7. *I've made so many mistakes* ("I've made too many mistakes to try anything new now").

8. *My husband (wife) would kill me* ("If I create things to look forward to, my family would say no, that it's not a good idea").

9. *I'm a quitter* ("I can't make plans because I always quit").

10. *I'm not psychologically equipped* ("I have so much anxiety and self-doubt that I don't believe I'm able to do something I always wanted to do").

11. *I'm not a religious person* ("I have no faith in anything with purpose and meaning so I don't believe it's in the cards for me to look forward to something").

12. *I have no hope* ("At this age I have nothing to be excited about. My life is almost over, and I can't imagine anything more for me").

13. *Having a dream house is too big a project* ("I hate my house but how can we up and move? We're settled in, and the thought of packing and moving is overwhelming.")

14. *My family would laugh at me* ("My kids see me as a grandmother, not as a 'jet set' person who can travel to explore the world").

15. *I have no spark* ("Doing something outrageous would exceed my oomph").

16. *My bones ache* ("How could I traipse around Europe when my legs and joints hurt").

17. *My wife is sick* ("My wife is sick. I'm her caretaker, and I can't look forward to something because she's dependent on me").

18. *I'm not spiritual* ("I'm not a glass-half-full kind of person, believing in stuff. I'm a realist").

19. *No one wants me* ("No way someone would want to be with me as a partner at this stage of my life").

Imagine That ONE Thing

Sure, life seems to have a way of dictating to us what we come to think of as our lot in this world, and we see no hope for such to change. Well, this couldn't be further from the truth. This collective list of reasons above stating we have nothing to look forward to is a short list. I could have filled the entire book with reasons people give as to why they have nothing to look forward to, but I didn't want to make this section a downer. Rather I want to offer an uplifter.

I want you to imagine that ONE thing you desire most, which could lie ahead for you in life — anything you like, whether or not others support you in this. Identifying that experience, that dream, that wish is a start to having something to look forward to. That ONE thing can be as simple as taking a walk along the beach every morning and becoming one with nature (through a forest, by a lake, in a park). Or that ONE thing can be planting flowers of any size, shape, and color, and clipping a few for a vase in your home for you to smell and appreciate.

Maybe you dreamt of becoming a teacher or a professor. Okay, you could adapt that dream, and you could tutor children in a local school, or read stories to the residents in a nursing home. That ONE thing can be anything you imagine it to be, and how you take that simple idea and make it work for you can be anything that strikes you as well. Don't worry about rules or boundaries as to how far your imagination can take you. And what we imagine, we can nudge into fruition.

Many times, effects we think we can't look forward to come about through confronting and accepting some seemingly uncomfortable change in ourselves. Maybe, for instance, you were taught to be selfless and that to want something to look forward to is a selfish act. You think you don't deserve and shouldn't want what you really do want—without realizing that the universe, your source, may well be inviting you there—wants you to want that. You can change your thinking on the subject, even if you have to mull over the idea for a while.

One way to find that ONE thing to look forward to is to look at what you're passionate about. A patient of mine, Arlene, told me she always wanted to be a painter, but that she didn't have "a stitch of artistic ability" in her. So, we imagined where this passion could carry her. We talked about adult coloring books, her taking art classes, joining an art group, but those seemed wrong to her somehow. Yet when we talked about her purchasing pieces she could paint herself—pieces already made that only required paining, she lit up. We had hit the jackpot. Her patio is now filled with her delightful painted sculptures that make her smile at every glance.

Another woman, Anna, in her late fifties, had some disabilities, but she didn't let them stand in her way. She joined a group of five other women, and weekly they meet together to paint pictures. They watch tutorials on painting, and then go to town copying the strategies to bring the art into realization.

Anna has many beautiful paintings in her home that she's proud of. In fact, I have one I'll cherish forever and ever. The picture is of a bridge surrounded by trees decorated by fresh peaks of newly dropped snow. The snow in the painting is picture perfect—you know, the stage when it's clean and white and new. I smile every day when I see that picture as it reminds me of a similar one I had many, many years before—and lost in a divorce. This painting is precious to me.

To look forward to something is about building a life filled with passion and excitement. You can look forward to writing your next non-fiction book or that great novel by starting it now—today. Why wait?

I think about a librarian, Darlene, who lost her job because libraries in the schools became obsolete—or the printer, Jake, who no longer was able to use the old time printing press, or the film developer, Arthur, who no longer had people coming in his store to develop film. Did they give up? No.

All were in their retirement years, but rather than quitting, each of them regrouped. Darlene, the librarian, now drives a fun-filled bus to the various schools to teach the children about reading. Jake, the printer, learned ways to digitally print. And the film developer, Arthur, turned his store into an art gallery with photos hanging on the walls. Ten small steps toward looking forward to the future years of your life can fulfill you in ways you never thought possible.

Ten Steps to Happy

1. **Don't Make Excuses.** We have plenty of time to look forward to something. Believe a beautiful outcome is possible, and watch the wonder appear. Start small with baby steps, and you'll build a life you look forward to in every waking moment.
2. **Have Ample Sleep.** Sleep is the key to your physical health. When you're sleeping, your body is healing and repairing. Studies show sleep deficiency is linked to increased risk of kidney disease, high blood pressure, diabetes, heart disease, and stroke, not to mention it will make you crabby and less able to concentrate and function in daily activities.
3. **Take the Leap.** Those who want their dreams to manifest are willing to take the risk. They don't look for the negative or allow the naysayers to knock down the dream. They push forward, and don't look back.

4. **Work toward Attainable Goals.** You want to make your goals achievable. Sometimes our thinking is cloudy, and we believe we can't have something, or that we're not worthy—I'm not talking about that. I'm talking about setting the goal realistically. For example, if you want to bike through parts of Italy, you have to start by getting into physical shape and assuring you have the finances to travel there. You can work with a trainer to ready yourself physically and save your money to afford the trip.

5. **Never Quit.** Winners never quit, and quitters never win. I remember this saying shared with me by a friend of mine in my college days. That helpful friend, Thomas Powers, caught me in a down time in my life and showed up at my doorstep holding a newspaper article with the quote: "Winners never quit and quitters never win." This was from the amazing football coach Vince Lombardi. I never forgot. I was in my early twenties.

6. **Remain Consistent.** To realize your dreams of things to look forward to, you need to be consistent with the dream. Cherish every opportunity you have to do what you love and do it well.

7. **Make the Best of Every Situation.** Life will come with some tough knocks. Perhaps people you love will die, become sick, or have terrible things happen to them—or you may be the one subject to illness or bad "luck." But, if you're going to power

through the good times and the bad, you must be ready and able to make the best of every situation, because tough times are sure to come. However, bad is always followed by good. Behind every cloud, the sun awaits.

8. **Take Responsibility for Your Life.** Don't wait for something to happen by chance, because that's like shooting a target in the dark. You'll miss the target. It's up to you to choose happy, to choose circumstances and events to look forward to. Use what you have, and what you know to make it happen.

9. **Cherish the Journey.** If you're always looking ahead at what you don't have, or what you don't have to look forward to, you're building this as your truth. Stop it. If you're going to succeed in having something to look forward to, you need self-discipline to make yourself do what you need to when you should do it, whether you feel like following through at the moment, or not.

10. **Stay Healthy.** If you want to do those fun things and have much to look forward to, you have to take *good* care of yourself. You must eat real food, include moderate exercise, drink lots of water, sleep sufficiently, and hang around with positive people, not naysayers.

As we come closer to winding down in this book I want to touch on the fact that we can't do this life alone, we need other people—people need people, plus fur and feather companions too. They are precious and innocent and loving and can teach us much, as you will see in Chapter 19.

Personal Inventory Questions

1. *It's never too late to be what you might have been.* ~George Eliot. What did you want to be?
2. If you had to pick that ONE thing you always wanted to do, what would it be?
3. My Great Great Aunt Mary Starks went into the military past the age of enlistment, even when others told her that wasn't possible. She made it happen, though all odds were against her as a woman, and older than the age to enlist. What relative inspired you? Why?
4. How did you receive the words of Dr. Dyer from *Your Erroneous Zones*: "The next time you are contemplating a decision in which you are debating whether or not to take charge of yourself, to make your own choice, ask yourself an important question, 'How long am I going to be dead?'" Sometimes harsh words shake us awake. Did this quote shake you out of not paying attention to making the most of your life?
5. Society has a way of dictating what we should or shouldn't be doing at a certain age, but the opinion of others isn't necessarily valid. Do you know someone who started a business, career, or degree at a later age? How did their journey affect you?

6. Wendy and Anthony both started other careers after retiring, but this time careers built on love and passion. Can you do the same? What's stopping you?

7. Okay, let's now focus on the reasons *you* aren't living your life with purpose — something to look forward to. What's blocking you? What are your excuses?

8. Imagine that ONE thing you really want for your future — anything you like, even if others don't support you. Imagine without any reservation that ONE thing you would do if you knew nothing or nobody would stand in your way? Dream big!

9. In the, *I have nothing to look forward to* list, which excuses did you circle? What negation of dreams do you have that aren't listed? How can you make such a list of your own positive rather than negative?

10. In the Ten Steps to Happy, which ones resonate with you? Can you make a personal additional ten steps to happy? What do your steps look like?

Chapter 19

People Need People

*The most wasted of all days
is one without laughter
~E.E. Cummings*

When was the last time you watched little kids giggling? Their entire bodies laugh to the point they may even fall to the ground. When was the last time you laughed like that? I recently read that laughter can increase oxygen and endorphins, improve your mood, and reduce physical pain. Now that's a big bang for a bit of a giggle. Think back to the last time you had one of those deep belly laughs; I bet just thinking about it makes you start to chuckle.

Did you know endorphins are the body's natural painkillers? And now you know that by laughing you could release these very endorphins, which help lighten chronic pain, hence making you feel good all over. But most of the time, we aren't laughing by ourselves; we're laughing with someone, or about something.

Yes, for the most part, laughter involves something or somebody to make us laugh. I bet for most of us, our spouse, children, grandchildren, other family members, beloved pet(s), and/or friends are the ones who bring about the giggles.

During the isolation time with the coronavirus, most of us realized more than ever, how important other people and our fur and feather children are.

I'll admit I can be a bit of a loner, as you read in the chapter "Extrovert Or Introvert?" but that's by choice. I've prided myself on the fact I'm entertained much of the time solely by myself with books and writing, along with long walks — but since the "imposed" isolation and social distancing, I'm missing people. I miss sitting face to face in person with my youngest son and his wife. I miss seeing patients in the flesh, not separated by a computer screen. I miss seeing smiles rather than mask coverings.

In fact, a dear friend of mine shared with me a blog by a psychiatrist friend that so spoke to me, and to this point, that people do need people:

"I spoke to an old therapist friend and finally understood why everyone's so exhausted after video calls. It's the plausible deniability of everyone's absence. Our

minds are tricked into the idea of being together when our bodies feel we're not. Dissonance is exhausting.

"It's easier being in each other's presence, or each other's absence, than in the constant presence of each other's absence. Our bodies process so much context, so much information, in encounters, that meeting on video is being a weird kind of blindfolded.

"We sense too little and can't imagine enough, that single deprivation requires a lot of effort." ~Gianpiero Petriglieri, INSEAD, Paris.

I was fascinated with Dr. Petriglieri's conclusions on video sessions, as I've been locked away for months and months seeing patients on this new platform, and feeling a sense something is missing. This medical doctor and psychiatrist, who now researches and practices leadership development, understands firsthand the importance of people needing people.

Too often these days we are separated from in-person gatherings by masks, computers, and phones, leaving most of us to feel lonely and isolated. And to the doctor's point, we are missing the natural gestures we can only see and feel in person. Having such distance from people on an ongoing basis, whether they are the ones we love or merely 'others,' isn't natural.

A Simple Smile

Back in my thirteen years of Weight Watchers days, I often paired up with a lovely woman named Beverly, who was more than twice my age, to lecture to large groups in business and hospital settings. We were quite a duo. Beverly was stunning — movie star-Grace Kelly (Princess of Monaco) stunning. And I was young and thirsty for knowledge that she freely gave.

Beverly had class and dignity, always. She spoke of youth to the crowd of thin-wanna-be's, encouraging them to eat healthy, exercise, drink loads of water, and smile — yes she'd say smile — and you'll lose ten years instantly without a facelift. She sparked a good laugh every time. She'd add to that the importance of rehydrating the skin through a simple glass of water. The message was drink lots and lots of water, and voila youthful skin, for sure. She'd go on about how you didn't need the fancy creams, surgeries, or other magical youth-promoting tactics, but rather to simply smile and drink water — both free.

Imagine laughter, smiles, and water all leading the way to youth, naturally. Imagine days, weeks, months, and years of being your best you, no matter your age.

How would you react waking up day after day, any place at any time in your life, and feeling good — really good, with your body, your face, your movement — all of it — being perfectly aligned with who you are as an individual, in all your endeavors.

People need people, unity, family, and conversation. While writing this book I was knee-deep in the pandemic and living in the epicenter of the virus. Jumping on a plane to see family stopped. Going out to dinner once in a while with my husband no longer took place. Seeing the smiles on people's faces was no longer possible as faces were covered in masks (rightfully) in every public place I went.

People DO need people. And as we age, we need people even more. We need that connection to feel whole and worthy. We need the connection to know others know we exist.

In *Mother Teresa: Reaching Out in Love*, a compilation of stories told by Mother Teresa, she recalled a group of teachers from the United States visiting India, who inquired, "Tell us something that will help us to live our lives better. What do you think we could do to bring peace and joy into the world?"

Now that's a huge question that might go all sorts of directions, but it didn't. Mother Teresa, with a big smile on her face, said: "Smile at each other. Smile at your husband, smile at your wife, smile at your children, be happy with your children. It doesn't matter who it is, smile at them."

Whoa, how simple is that? My goodness if a smile can bring peace and joy into the world—and as Beverly (who I spoke of earlier) says, it can make us look years younger—this smile thing is good.

And you wouldn't smile alone, unless you're having a memory of something; for the most part, you're smiling with another. People need people. And you can add your fur and feather kids to the mix too. Studies show animals DO experience a rich array of emotions, especially for their human family members.

This morning, I was driving from the east coast of Florida to the west coast of Florida with Oliver my

Eclectus parrot and Southern Grace, my white Swiss shepherd. We were set for a long weekend getaway, just the three of us. All the while, Oliver, who is always settled way in the back of my SUV so he can look out the window, was chatting: "Hello, oh wow, hello, I see you, hello, I love you" with a whistle and giggle here and there. And then Miss Grace nuzzled my ear from time to time when she wasn't poking her head out the window, taking in the fresh air and fitting in barking at the car inching up beside us. And meanwhile I was smiling, feeling totally connected to them — totally blessed, in the moment.

Between your pets and people, you can find ways to foster a deeper connection. How? you may ask. Well by getting out and doing something with someone or your pet. Don't sit idle and alone for long periods of time. By becoming involved and doing more than not, you'll feel younger than you did ten years ago. People who don't fret over numbers or what other people think, and connect with others, seem almost ageless.

Don't become caught in a rut where you're doing the same thing day in and day out, without stimulation. Call a friend and go for a walk, or join that gym you've been thinking for years about joining. Or, how about participating in a book club with like-minded people — or perhaps not like-minded, to hear another point of view.

Or what about Events and Adventures, founded almost thirty years ago, which offers fun events to attend, such as wine tastings or operas, but also has

311

very active gatherings like jet skiing, glass blowing, and spelunking (exploring caves). Though a cost is involved, this is a way to meet people in an organized group kind of setting.

Or maybe you always wanted to cruise through Europe, or bike through Italy, or discover the streets of Paris; you'll find groups you can do this with. As we grow older, seeking novel experiences and challenging ourselves may not come naturally to us. We become more fearful with the unknowns and what ifs.

We may be set in a pattern and revert back to it over and over, without finding our way out of the same loop. In our younger years going here and there without thinking about physical risks was easier, but that's not so as we get on. We know better, based on past experiences, whereas the young take the plunge without thinking of possible consequences.

Perhaps our goals shift some as well once we move into our middle age and beyond, causing us to prioritize emotional stability and meaningful experiences and relationships. That's a good thing. We're more selective and what we do tends to be more from the heart. All good.

No matter the age, stepping out of our comfort zones may be challenging, but it does become less risky mentally as we move on in age. As we progress beyond our earlier years, we rise in confidence and are more stable, based on all the scrapes and bruises we endured and overcame along the way.

Older people report being more emotionally stable, and happy and content as well as less affected by negative events, because as time goes on, we do become better at managing our emotions, and worry less about what others might think.

So as you power through with people and pets in mind, take on something new every day. Try a small change like taking a bath instead of a shower, walk in another direction than the usual, join a friend for dinner rather than eating alone. If your friend(s) lives far away, (a next best to in person) then connect through Zoom or Facetime or whatever other digital connection you have and you'll find you're not feeling as alone. The point is to do something new you haven't done before, or that's not part of your routine.

Find people who inspire and encourage you. Stay away from the malcontent persons, especially ones who are chronically discontented or dissatisfied with life. And hug…yes hug people. Okay, if we're still in the pandemic, you might not want to be hugging strangers, but I pray by the time this book is out, the virus will be behind us – and we can touch again.

Sexually Connect

No matter the age, sex is an important ingredient to wholeness. Often couples stop engaging because life turns so busy with the kids and career that sex falls by the wayside. Or perhaps illness or sexual malfunction has stepped in the way. No matter the reason, intimacy and connection are *still* important later in

313

life. For most of us, the two greatest joys in life are our kids and career, but as the years go by, the kids are grown and flown, and the career may slow down or completely stop. Now what? Now you have two once-intimate people disconnected.

But the relationship's not over; so here you have an opportunity to reconnect as adults, without the children or the busyness of work. Fear not, you can have a healthy, rewarding sex life, at any age. If a while has gone by without that kind of closeness, start easy by dating your partner. Yes, dating. When was the last time you held hands and took a stroll?

Whether you and your partner have been going through a dry spell or you're beginning fresh with someone new, you can ignite the flame. When was the last time you looked deeply into each other's eyes the way you used to, and shared a dream or a wish? Start slow.

According to *Help Guide* (helpguide.org), a guide to mental health and wellness, sex can be a powerful emotional experience and a great tool for protecting or improving health. And sex isn't only for the young. The need for intimacy is felt by all ages. The site's article goes on to say that studies now confirm no matter your gender, you can enjoy sex for as long as you wish.

For sure, sexual relations at our older years will not be the same as they were in our twenties or thirties—but they can be equally as satisfying, and perhaps maybe even better. As we mature, and as we become more confident and wiser, we engage our loved one with trust and intimacy at a higher, deeper level. This is so because we are more self-confident, with self-awareness and aren't seeking to fill unrealistic goals.

The article goes on to promote the benefits of sex as we age to improve mental and physical health, increase life span, solidify relationships, and provide emotional refuge.

Steps to a Later Love Life

How can we improve our romantic lives in older age? Here are some ideas, below.

- **Become Acquainted:** Spend time together to find out what one another's dreams and hopes are. Learn what makes your partner feel safe and comfortable.
- **Practice Mindfulness:** Sometimes the head talk clouds the moment. Shut down your head chatter by becoming more present in the now.
- **Be Playful:** Intimate relations don't have to be confined to the bedroom. Perhaps you have a pool that offers privacy or you can create a fun environment in a different room in your home.
- **Set the Scene:** Put on some quiet music, perhaps something without lyrics, but rather a melody that can sweep you into a relaxed state. Remember to set the lighting to your needs and add fresh sheets and scents.
- **Discuss New Ideas:** As we age, we may have to find more creative ways to make love. Be

open-minded and consider the opportunity to use mechanical help.

- **Rewire Your Attitude:** Leave your negative self out of the bedroom, and let go of the sex of yesterday so you can surrender to the sex of today.
- **Love Your Body:** Give gratitude and thanks for your body, every inch of it. Take the time to groom and brush your teeth and wash to create a beautiful partner for your other.
- **Renew Your Sexy:** Find a lovely nightgown, night attire, or robe that you feel attractive wearing.

Ten Steps To a Healthier You

As we near the finish line, I want to leave you with some simple yet profound tips for guidance to cultivating a healthy body and mind. Be sure you don't make this your "To Do" list because then these ideas become a chore, not a fun ten steps to a healthier you.

1. **Eat Real Food:** No doubt by now you know food is a great start to putting together a healthier you. Eat real food to fuel your body and your mind.
2. **Write an Achievement List:** Sometimes we forget how much we've accomplished in life, minimizing our successes. Write out your achievement list. At this stage of our lives we may feel less useful, forgetting what we've attained. You've brought forth so much—go as far back as you need to. I

pulled out my old yearbook at my 45th reunion and didn't realize all the credentials I'd earned. I thought I was a loser.

3. **Design a Vision Board:** Create a vision board mapping out your upcoming intentions. Vision boards are a powerful way to shift your mindset into future plans by visualizing and creating the life you want. Let go, be creative—a vision board has no boundaries. Make sure to put your vision board where you can see it day in and day out, reminding you of what your dreams are. You are subconsciously manifesting your future and growing all your accomplishments merely going through the work of putting together your vision of you.

4. **Become Grounded:** Earthing, which we spoke of in Chapter 15, is a way to connect to the earth and to your Higher Source. Take off your shoes and put your feet in the grass, feel the earth.

5. **Schedule "Me" Time:** Schedule time for you. Make an appointment with yourself, whether to write, read, or take a nap. Checking in with self and taking some time to be quiet is important—or maybe for you the schedule isn't about being quiet but to connect with people.

6. **Find a Soul Tribe:** Create or find a soul tribe or a community you connect with. I personally have a few writing groups I hang with, along with dog people, psychology groups, and my online friends to fill my soul with the like-minded. Step out of

your comfort zone and discover people you can connect with. People really do need people.

7. **Commit:** Do you know what you're going to do when you commit, what you'll actually accomplish? When I was coming out of my food addiction, I wrote my food down every single day without fail for seven years and initially, for four years, sent it to my sponsor, and then to myself for another three years, totaling seven years. Writing this down committed me to my plan and the way of life I live to this day—seventeen-plus years later.

8. **Express Gratitude:** Make a gratitude list. I wrote about creating a gratitude list at length in my second book, *Release Your Obsession with Diet Chatter, Heal from the Inside Out.* Making such a list helped me through some very dark days and continues to refresh my ability to see reasons to be grateful.

9. **Use Positive Mantras:** Create positive statements or slogans, and repeat frequently. A helpful book I have used was Louise Hay's book on this, *Experience Your Good Now! Learning to Use Affirmations.* I would write out an affirmation daily and post it on my computer screen and phone screen, and recorded it to listen to. One that comes to mind: "I am strong and bountiful and positive, and I move through very difficult times every time, even when I think I can't."

10. **Use Your Intuition:** Trust your inner voice that lets you know with a nudge if you're on the right track. Often, we ignore and push away the hunch. Don't do that. We need our inner cues to guide us. When I planned to write my first book, *Release Your Obsession with Food: Heal from the Inside Out*, I was scared, but inside I knew for years this was what I was supposed to do — write. I didn't look at the cost or time it would take, I just plunged forward one word at a time. Oh sure, sometimes I feared the book might not be received well, but a wise author once said, "Write for yourself." And I have done that since.

We will next turn our attention to the last chapter: Final Thoughts.

Personal Inventory Questions

1. It's true: *The most wasted of all days is the one without laughter* (E.E. Cummings). Do you laugh daily? Think back to the last time you laughed, who was with you, and what was happening. I bet thinking about it makes you laugh — or at least smile.

2. People DO need people. Who are the people in your life, and how do they fill you? If negative, regroup and corral people who add to your life, filling your cup with positive.

3. I recently read that laughter can increase oxygen and endorphins, improve your mood, and reduce physical pain. Do you believe this to be true, or a bunch of hogwash? The next time you're in pain, or perhaps even now while you're reading this,

laugh and watch the pain disappear as you kick up those endorphins.

4. Perhaps you feel more alive and youthful around animals. Recall the last time you felt happy and alive with your fur/feather kid. What was going on? How did the relationship make you feel?

5. Maybe your friends live far away. Did you ever consider connection through a video chat? Maybe you feel this is too techy, but I assure you, any little person in your life can teach you, and you'll be connected in a nanosecond.

6. Sex is not just for the young adult—it's for you too, no matter your age. Be creative. Make a list of comfortable actions you can take for a romantic time with your significant other.

7. Think about the last time you engaged with an animal. What was your experience? Did it make you laugh? Are you smiling now just thinking about it?

8. Where would you like to go? Can you think of a place you've dreamt of visiting? What has kept you from going? List some possible ways to make this dream come true.

9. Sometimes we forget how much we've accomplished, minimizing our impact on the world. At this stage of our lives, we may feel less useful. Write out an achievement list.

10. Who have you been thinking about lately? Pick up the phone and call that person. Make a way to connect.

Chapter 20

Final Thoughts

As we are liberated from our own fear,
Our presence automatically liberates others
~ Marianne Williamson

In late November, under a crisp, gray-slated sky, only days before Thanksgiving, I briskly made my way through the Chicago O'Hare International Airport, fearing I'd miss my flight home to South Florida, as I was running late. A handsome, young rock'n roll kinda guy caught my eye as he moved swiftly through the crowds as well. A deep-brown leather backpack was strapped on his shoulders, complementing the washed-out blue jeans with rips purposely placed, and a caramel-colored t-shirt. His long, wavy, velvet-black hair was blowing in the man-made breeze, as he raced to catch his plane. Our eyes met.

My thought was *What a good-looking guy. Must be in a band.* He had *that look* and that smell of mint mixed with rose and cinnamon, Paco Rabanne, I'd guessed, as the scent wafted in my direction. But soon I forgot about the *GQ* hunk and moved on to check in my luggage and wait to board.

The plane was crowded, and I was one of the last to find my seat. I climbed over the woman in the aisle seat bundled in her winter coat, scarf, and boots, thrilled that the window seat was still vacant, hoping it would stay that way so I could scoot over and stretch out. But soon one last stroller sprinted down the aisle, stopping smack at our row. We each stood to let in *Mr. Paco Rabanne.*

As he plunked deep into his seat, I noted he was sniffing, as if he really needed to blow his nose — to the extent that he began wiping it on his shirt for lack of a napkin or Kleenex. Of course. I continued profiling, this time concluding he was definitely a rock'n roller *on cocaine.* Through the entire flight, he sniffed, coughed, put his head down on the tray — then back on the headrest, desperately trying to make himself comfortable.

Mr. *GQ* was flushed and sweating, completely present with his distress. At one point, as I began to drift off into much needed sleep, he bounced up, saying, "I have to get out, I have to get out!" And once again the woman on the aisle and I rose backing up to let him prance down the walkway between the sections of the seats, making his way to the bathroom.

I'd barely placed my head on my little pillow before he was climbing in again, and I blurted out, "Damn that was fast!" He looked startled, and several people laughed.

Just in the nick of time, the plane landed in Ft. Lauderdale, and off I went—and Paco Rabanne as well, with his backpack slung over his shoulders, walking with a slight drag to his step, and looking as though he'd seen better days. The guy had disintegrated right before my eyes from being the hot guy at the airport in Chicago to the hollow-eyed, bedraggled one in Florida. And soon I forgot him as he walked off and I headed for home.

Well, my seatmate was forgotten until Wednesday that was, two days later, and one day before Thanksgiving, when I began to come down with a fierce sore throat, sniffles, and a wicked cough, and felt as if I couldn't breathe. I went to work but struggled through my day with cough drops, hot tea, tons of tissues, and refills of water. I felt achy everywhere and just plain awful, all rolled into one. And then...*the hunk came to mind*. I realized he was not the cokehead he had seemed to be, but rather a very, very unwell young man.

And now, so was I very, very ill. I remained sick for months with constant relapses—but never missed work. Several times, I suggested to my husband that I might need to go to the hospital because my chest hurt with a sensation that felt like a combination of pressure and prickling. This went on from November all the way to the start of February. And I don't ever come down with something.

No, I never went to the hospital because every time I thought I might or maybe I'd go to a walk-in clinic, I'd start to feel better before I'd relapse again. I'm not one to run to the doctor, as I'm healthy—really healthy. And each time I thought I might go at least to the walk-in clinic, the next day I'd seem much better. My body was so healthy from the start that it was pushing out this illness, and then the infection would fight to stick with me—until it was finally gone, with the exception of low energy and respiratory challenges to date, yes, to now, so many months later.

As we are liberated from our own fears, our presence automatically liberates others, as Marianne Williamson states.

I NEVER become sick, and I mean never. I pride myself on eating healthy, exercising, meditating, and living life as if it's a prayer. So much for that! I became fearful I had something really wrong, some deep illness. And then, soon to follow, the pandemic hit America—this faraway illness that I first heard about coming from Wuhan, China. Did I have this coronavirus, I pondered, along with so many others?

I began writing this book about tackling the obsession with aging in a healthy and excited state, never imagining directly in the middle of my writing I'd be in the center of a worldwide COVID-19 pandemic. My quest to build a positive view on aging was knocked wide open with a virus—and I think I might have caught it from the cutie-pie on the plane.

No doubt, adverse events occur even when you live your best life physically, emotionally, and spiritually. I shudder to think what might have happened had I not lived a healthy life; perhaps I wouldn't be here today. So as I edge closer to 64 years of age, I'm feeling strong, laced with vitality and energy once again. We all age, and we all die, though the journey doesn't have to be dire—but rather can be an opportunity for aging with dignity.

Life would be much simpler if we were all born with a book that told us how to age gracefully, a book that answered our deepest internal fears and gave us the go-ahead that it's okay to age, a book that delivered support when we needed it. But in the end, we must all write this book for ourselves and find our true path in life as it unfolds.

This gift is in each of us—it is not the outside that speaks to our souls—our inner beings—but rather what is within.

The end result I've tried to produce in *Release Your Obsession With Aging: Heal from the Inside Out* is a blend of a spiritual slant on aging obsessions, together with practical, down-to-earth advice. My goal has been to help you learn how to live more fully day to day in order to break from a negative, compulsive, self-destructive mentality (or any form of self-degradation or a *just for today* attitude) no matter where you are, who you're with, or what situation is at hand. I hope I accomplished at least a portion of this grand task.

*****

I have one final request before I leave you, at least for now before you check out my other books on Obsessions. If you can spare me just a few moments, can you please leave a few words of wisdom so prospective readers can better understand if they will find inspiration in this book or not. Many thanks in advance!! Dr. Lisa

Acknowledgements

This book represents a personal inquiry into a confusing aspect of my own experience. As I began to make sense out of unexpected changes in my life, patients with the same needs emerged. This ultimately led to my writing about my discoveries, to share with others in similar situations.

No book is written without the contributions of many people. My wish is to recognize every spoken and unspoken inspired word, but I don't have enough pages, so regrettably I can only mention a few.

I wouldn't have written about these things if not for my husband, Joe, who encourages me to follow my dreams, no matter how small or how large they may be. Also, I thank my sons, Kris and Benjamin, who have always been a source of help with technical, legal, and administrative tasks beyond my comprehension. And I must mention with gratitude my beloved parents, Benjamin and Joan, who shine down from heaven, prompting me to continue to move forward in my efforts to help those with similar challenges to the ones I faced.

No book can sing without a great editor, which goes without saying. My editor, G. Miki Hayden, is a godsend. This is our fourth book together, and we have become quite a team. She miraculously breathes life into this mission of mine to help others make peace with the obsessions within many of us. G.

Miki's suggested edits also struck a chord with me and helped me move out of the way of the work at hand, shaping and rounding it into a true journey.

Last, a huge shout-out to ALL my patients over the past twenty-three years, who taught and continue to teach me. Thank you from my heart!

Bibliography

American Psychiatric Association. (2013). *Diagnostic and Statistical Manual of Mental Disorders (5th ed.).* Arlington, VA: American Psychiatric Association Publishing.

Borysenko, J. (1996). *A Woman's Book Of Life: The Biology, Psychology, and Spirituality of the Feminine Life Cycle.* New York, NY. Riverhead Books.

Bulut, E.A., Khoury, R. Lee, H. & Grossberg, G. (2019). Eating Disturbances in the Elderly: A Geriatric-Psychiatric Perspective. *Journal of Nutrition and Healthy Aging,* Vol.5, no.3, pp.185-198.

Cahalan, S. (2012). *Brain on Fire.* New York, NY: Simon & Schuster.

Carlson, R. (1997). *You Can Be Happy No Matter What: Five Principles Your Therapist Never Told You.* Novato, CA: New World Library.

Covey, S. (1990). *The 7 Habits of Highly Effective People: Powerful Lessons in Personal Change.* New York, NY: First Fireside Edition, Simon and Schuster.

Dyer. W. (1976). *Your Erroneous Zones: Step-by-Step Advice for Escaping the Trap of Negative Thinking and Taking Control of Your Life.* New York: Funk & Wagnalls.

Fonda, J. (2006). *My Life So Far*. New York: Random House.

Furnham, A., Levitas, J. (2012). Factors that Motivate People to Undergo Cosmetic Surgery. *The Canadian Journal of Plastic Surgery, 20(4): e47-e50*. Retrieved on March 14, 2020 from https://bit.ly/3kdppTU.

Jantz, G. with McMurray, A. (2003). *Moving Beyond Depression: A Whole Person Approach to Healing*. Colorado Springs, Colorado: WaterBrook Press.

Haddock, K. & Dill, P. (2000). The effects of food on mood and behavior: Implications for the addictions model of obesity and eating disorders. *Hawthorne Press Inc., 15* (1), 17-47.

Harvard's Men's Health Watch (2016). *Preserve Your Muscle Mass*. Harvard Health Publishing Retrieved on March 29, 2020 from https://www.health.harvard.edu/staying-healthy/preserve-your-muscle-mass .

Hay, L. (2012). *You Can Heal Your Life*. Carlsbad, Ca.: Hay House Publishers.

Hill, S. (2019). *Dangerous Prayers: 50 Powerful Prayers that Changed the World*. Nashville, Tennessee: Thomas Nelson.

Kubler-Ross, E. (1969). *Death and Dying.* New York: Macmillan Publishing Co. Inc.

Lama, D. & Chan V. (2004). *The Wisdom of Forgiveness: Intimate Conversations and Journeys.* New York, NY: Riverhead Books

Le Joly, E. & Chaliha, J. (1998). *Mother Teresa's Reaching Out in Love.* New York, NY: Barns and Noble.

Lightman, A. (2020). *In Praise of Wasting Time.* New York: Simon and Schuster.

Lipton, B. (2015). *The Biology of Belief: Unleashing the Power of Consciousness, Matter & Miracles.* Carlsbad, Ca.: Hay House Publishers.

Moore, B. (2004). *Believing God.* Nashville, Tennessee: Broadman & Holman Publishers.

Osteen, J. (2011). *Every Day A Friday: How To Be Happier 7 Days A Week.* New York, NY: Faith Works.

OWN (2020). Oprah and Jennifer Lopez: Your Life in Focus. Retrieved on March 23, 2020 from Oprah's Super Soul Conversations: OWN.

Ortigara Crego, L. (2017*). Release Your Obsession with Food: Heal from the Inside Out.* Hollywood, Florida: Madeira Publishing.

Ortigara Crego, L. (2018). *Release Your Obsession with Diet Chatter: Heal from the Inside Out.* Hollywood, Florida: Madeira Publishing.

Ortigara Crego, L. (2019). *Release Your Obsession with Cheat DAZE: Heal from the Inside Out.* Hollywood, Florida: Madeira Publishing.

Pettinger, T. (2006). *Biography Mother Teresa.* Biography Online, Retrieved on June 15, 2020 from https://www.biographyonline.net/nobelprize/mother_teresa.html .

Ramsey, D. (2003). *The Total Money Makeover: A Proven Plan for Financial Fitness.* Nashville, Tennessee: Thomas Nelson, Inc.

Rankin, H. (2019). *I Think Therefore I Am Wrong: A Guide to Bias, Political Correctness, Fake News and the Future of Mankind.* Howard J. Rankin, PhD.

Rosenzweig, M., Breedlove, S., & Leiman, A. (2002). *Biological Psychology: An Introduction to Behavioral, Cognitive, and Clinical Neuroscience.* Sunderland, Massachusetts: Sinauer Associates, Inc. Publishers.

Rogers, F. (2019). *A Beautiful Day in the Neighborhood: Neighborly Words of Wisdom from Mister Rogers.* New York: Penguin Books.

Sallah, M. & Perez, M. (2019). This Business Helped Transform Miami Into a National Plastic Surgery Destination. Eight Women Died. *USA Today* and *Naples Daily News*. Retrieved on March 21, 2020 from: https://bit.ly/2J7XMvz .

Shmerling, R.H. *Showering daily – is it necessary?* Retrieved on June 13, 2020 from Harvard Health Blog, posted June 26, 2019, https://bit.ly/2UE5bsr .

Smith,M. & Segal, J. (2019). *Better Sex as You Age.* Help Guide: Your Trusted Guide to Mental Health & Wellness. Retrieved on June 27, 2020 from: https://www.helpguide.org/articles/alzheimers-dementia-aging/better-sex-as-you-age.htm .

Siegel, B. (1993). *How to Live Between Office Visits: A Guide to Life, Love, and Health.* New York, NY: Harper Collins Publisher.

Weiss, B. (1988). *Many Lives, Many Masters: The True Story of a Prominent Psychiatrist, His Young Patient and the Past-Life Therapy That Changed Both their Lives.* New York: Fireside.

Young, L. (2019). *Remove Obstacles to Experience Unstoppable Feminine Power: How to Stop Betraying Yourself and Live a Life of Grace and Passion.* Laura B. Young, Publisher.

About the Author

Dr. Ortigara Crego, a clinical psychotherapist, addiction psychologist, and visiting professor in private practice, has worked in the field of eating disorders for well over two-and-a-half decades. She earned a doctorate in addiction psychology and a Master's degree in social work with the emphasis on mental health, and is certified as an eating disorder specialist, Master's certified addiction professional, and national board certified clinical hypnotherapist.

Dr. Ortigara Crego worked in the weight-loss industry for well over two decades. She speaks and blogs on recovery from compulsive/obsessive behaviors using spiritual and mind approaches to healing. She is the author of *Release Your Obsession with Food: Heal from the Inside Out*, a groundbreaking book on recovering from compulsive eating and spiritual deficits; *Release Your Obsession with Diet Chatter: Heal from the Inside Out*, a much needed book on quieting the drunken mental monkeys once and for all; and *Release Your Obsession from Cheat DAZE: Heal from the Inside Out*, a further exploration of the obsessions that affect those with food and other addictions. She contributed several chapters to SAGE Publications' Volume 1 and Volume 2 of the *Encyclopedia of Obesity* and runs a blog at Weightcontroltherapy.com.

Dr. Ortigara Crego's professional affiliations include the National Association of Social Workers, the National Board for Certified Clinical Hypnotherapists, the International Association of Eating Disorder Professionals, and the American Psychological Association.

Stay in Touch!

Please contact me at
<u>drlisaort@weightcontroltherapy.com</u>.

I would love to hear from you and learn from your experiences. Stop by my website:
http://weightcontroltherapy.com
to see what I'm up to and where I'm speaking next, along with what books I have planned, such as the next in the Release Your Obsession series, *Release Your Obsession with Money: Heal from the Inside Out.*

You can also find me on Facebook:
http://www.facebook.com/Drlisaortigaracrego
and on Twitter http://www.twitter.com/Drlisort and on Instagram http://www.Instagram.com/Drlisaort where we can engage in lively discussions on topics of health, including mental, physical, and spiritual wellbeing.

Made in the USA
Monee, IL
12 January 2021